ETHICAL ISSUES IN THE 21ST CENTURY

MISCONDUCT IN MEDICAL RESEARCH AND PRACTICE

ETHICAL ISSUES IN THE 21ST CENTURY

Additional books and e-books in this series can be found on Nova's website under the Series tab.

ETHICAL ISSUES IN THE 21ST CENTURY

MISCONDUCT IN MEDICAL RESEARCH AND PRACTICE

SERGEI V. JARGIN

nova science publishers
New York

NOTICE TO THE READER

Library of Congress Cataloging-in-Publication Data

ISBN: 978-1-53618-510-2

Published by Nova Science Publishers, Inc. † New York

CONTENTS

PREFACE

The main varieties of scientific misconduct are fabrication, falsification, misquoting and plagiarism. Considering the "improvement" of fraudulent skills, scientists, editors, and authorities must jointly combat the misconduct. Also, it is important that whistleblowers must be protected from revenge. The response to scientific misconduct requires national and international bodies to provide leadership and guidelines. Whistleblowers need a safe, confidential place to report misconduct. The quality of research and hidden conflicts of interest should be taken into account deciding which studies are to be included into reviews. Forged publications and speculative theories have been used for promotion of drugs, dietary supplements and treatments without proven effectiveness. Marketing of placebos in the guise of evidence-based medications seems to be on the increase. Patients can be misinformed not only by the advertising but also by publications supposed to be scientific. Furthermore, it has become usual practice to disregard published criticism in spite of personal communications and debates at conferences. Some scientists seem to make use of critical comments without citing them, or just continue publications ignoring the criticism. The same scientists continue working sometimes in cooperation with renowned researchers; and it is possible that some later articles are more reliable than earlier ones. However, it is insufficient to hope that reliable publications would be shortly confirmed while forgeries would fall into oblivion. Fake papers are misleading for research and practice, cost time and money. Wrong concepts are persisting and reappearing, which may result in useless experimentation and application of invasive methods without sufficient indications. An international cooperation of bona fide scientists, editors and authorities is needed to eradicate the scientific misconduct and fraude in medicine. The book contains an overview of misconduct in medical research and practice mainly from the former Soviet Union. Ample documentary evidence is provided as illustrations.

Sergei V. Jargin
Peoples' Friendship University of Russia

Chapter 1

THE BACKGROUND

The main varieties of scientific misconduct are well known: fabrication, falsification, misquoting and plagiarism (Figure 1.1). Besides, there are many subtypes and borderline violations: biased selection of data or specimens, discarding of "inconvenient" data, selective citation, "second hand" quotation without reading the article [1-3], citation of non-professional publications and commercial editions passing them off as scientific sources [4], publications without approval of the text by all co-authors, gift or honorary authorship, nepotism and companionship with mutual cover-up; violations of the rules of polemics, evasion from constructive discussion and questions at conferences, tangling of scientific texts and presentations, making them incomprehensible. The topic of scientific misconduct should not be exaggerated as it can throw suspicion on medicine and science in general. As far as reasonably possible, inquiries should be performed inside institutions without excessive publicity. Supposed perpetrators must be heard. Each new case of research misconduct must be investigated [5]. Admittedly, in some regions such as the former Soviet Union, where scientific misconduct has been widespread, excessively rigorous measures would more likely be destructive than constructive. Under these circumstances, the self-criticism with retraction of unreliable publications should be encouraged [6].

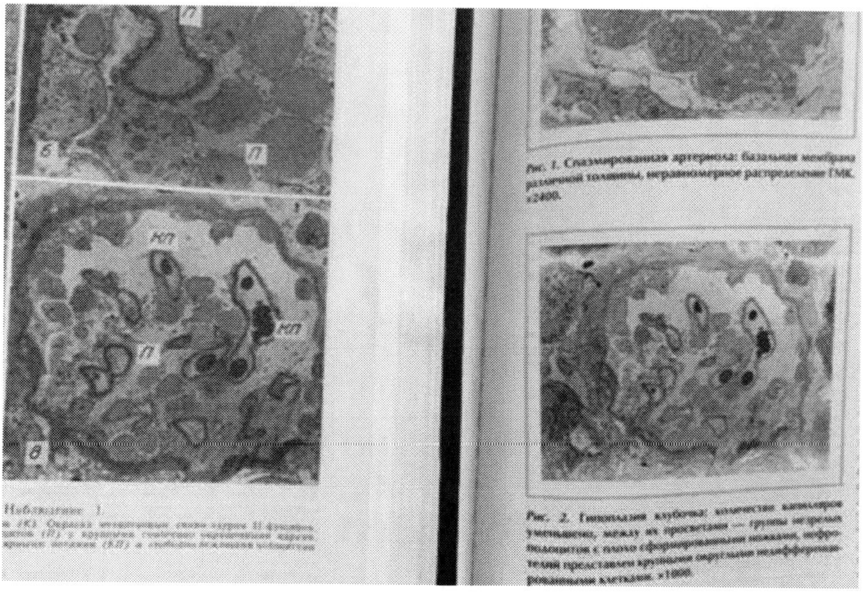

Figure 1.1. The same image published 25 years apart by different authors [7, 8]. Translation of the caption: glomerulus with singular capillary loops and freely lying podocytes X 1100 [7]. Comment: this is probably a tangential section of a normal renal glomerulus.

Furthermore, it has become usual practice to disregard published criticism in spite of personal communications and debates at conferences. Some scientists seem to make use of critical comments without citing them, or just continue publications ignoring the criticism. The same scientists continue working sometimes in cooperation with renowned researchers; and it is possible that some later articles are more reliable than earlier ones. However, it is insufficient to hope that reliable publications would be shortly confirmed while forgeries would fall into oblivion. Fake papers are misleading for research and practice, cost time and money. Wrong concepts are persisting and reappearing, which may result in useless experimentation and application of invasive methods without sufficient indications [9-11].

The fraudulent skills are improving: some scientific writers have perfected themselves in tangling their texts, making evaluation increasingly difficult. Scientific misconduct also includes measures against whistleblowers i.e., persons informing authorities on the fraud or publishing critical comments. The denunciation has been often condemned in the former Soviet Union; the fact of denunciation and the informer identity sometimes became known to other people including perpetrators with undesirable consequences for the whistleblowers up to a dismissal etc. Certain experts having criticized forged reports were exposed to mobbing and later dismissed [12]. The bullying of whistleblowers may continue also after a dismissal, in the place of residence and in other settings; some of them live in conditions of occasional violence and threats [13]. Whistleblowers must be protected from retaliation, need a safe, confidential venue to report misconduct [14]. It is not surprising that dishonest science flourishes under the conditions of corruption and priority of commercial interests over ethics. An important factor contributing to the misconduct is a hidden conflict of interest. Forged publications and speculative theories have been used for promotion of drugs, dietary supplements and treatments without proven effectiveness. Patients can be misinformed not only by the advertising but also by publications supposed to be scientific. Marketing of placebos in the guise of evidence-based medications seems to be on the increase [15].

Duplicate submissions and publications are also regarded as scientific misconduct. However, these acts are not related to the distortion of scientific truth and misappropriation of achievements. This "smaller evil" can be unavoidable thanks to editors, who are sometimes shelving important articles for long time, giving to the author no notice whether the manuscript will be published or not. Formally, the first submission must be withdrawn prior to a second submission of the same material, but it can be a suboptimal solution if the goal is a rapid publication and maximum resonance for the sake of scientific truth and public benefit. A delay can range from months to infinity. Certainly, it can be always objected that a peer review needs time. The responsibility may be with a reviewer delaying his or her comments (reviewer tardiness) [16-18] or with an author of a commented article, delaying a reply to a letter to the editor. A considerable delay of a decision about an important manuscript can be seen as a justification for a duplicate submission.

Inappropriate acts in the publication process committed by authors (plagiarism, misquoting, ghost or honorary authorship, hidden conflicts of interest, etc.) are well known. Less frequently discussed is an overt or disguised misconduct by editors. Among other things, editors must select competent and unbiased reviewers assuring that the decision about publication would be based solely on scientific qualities of the paper. Confidentiality must be maintained throughout the review process. Violations of these principles are difficult to prove, although suspicions that a reviewer is biased sometimes arise. Another problem is the copyediting of accepted manuscripts performed by some editors. The copyediting may improve the grammar and style; but in some cases it distorts the original meaning and imparts awkwardness, thus indirectly discrediting the author and/or the message of his article. How should the author react? If an accidental error seems to be probable, the matter can be discussed per e-mail and corrections carried out. When there are reasons to suspect a malicious intent, a discussion may be both disappointing and useless. Sometimes corrections are made but other text passages or references are concomitantly modified [18]. The motives are not always clear. There are suspicions that some auxiliary personnel, insufficiently controlled by editors, may be acting in accordance with interests of a third party trying to discredit the author, to impart awkwardness (e.g., [19]) or to make the author formally responsible for wrong statements [20] or misquoting. Making every effort to publish an important article, an author may see no alternative as to agree to a distorted version, or to make only essential corrections disregarding awkwardness of the copyedited text.

Paid open access publications are another topic: some publishers promise per e-mail a free publication; but later the author receives an invoice or payment requests from another e-mail address and contact person e.g., “financial department”. Inappropriate acts by some editors can be not only harmful for research and practice but also undermine international trust.

Finally, the publication of unserious abstracts in proceedings of international conferences should be mentioned, some of them commented in [21]. In the author’s opinion, the publication process and motives behind decisions should become more transparent. The response to misconduct in medical research and practice needs national and international bodies to provide leadership and guidelines [14], while the international cooperation of bona fide scientisis is of importance. In Russia, there is a Higher Attestation Commission, generally known as VAK, the main purpose of which is maintenance of a high level of scientific research. The VAK awards or approves of all academic degrees. Nevertheless, there are dissertations (theses) with detectable trimming of data, manipulations with statistics, misquoting, etc.; examples are in subsequent chapters. Official requirements to a doctoral thesis are difficult to comply with: it must be a "new large-scale scientific achievement or solution of a big scientific problem" (according to the governmental ordinance on the order of awarding of scientific degrees issued in 2002). In the preceding (1995) version of the ordinance there was a formulation: “Considerable contribution to the acceleration of scientific and technological advance”. Such requirements can move researchers towards strained interpretations at least. Other requirements applied both to doctoral and candidate dissertations are the global novelty and, in medicine, practical significance, which may be conducive to unfounded recommendations for the practice.

Another ingrained habit is the so-called “raisin”: modern methods expected to be applied in medical dissertations. As a result, modern methods are sometimes used without relevance, to enable claiming a “modern scientific level”. Another requirement to the doctoral dissertation is that main results must be published in peer-reviewed journals or editions officially acknowledged to be equivalent to them. As a result, scientific journals are overloaded by dubious and useless papers, while valuable manuscripts have to wait longer. Some functionaries have not enough time to prepare their dissertations and order them, or at least reviews of literature, from businesspeople offering such services. This is probably the cause of extensive misquoting found in some dissertations. An example provided here is the doctoral thesis (dissertation) of the chancellor of the First Moscow Medical University (previously named I.M. Sechenov Medical Academy) since 2010 [22]. The following illustrations are copies from the thesis [22] (Figure 1.2,3). Many authors’ names present in the text are absent in the reference list, which is a form of misquoting, some authors' names are misspelled. Some references presented on (Figure 1.3) were checked in the PubMed. Results:

Ref. 55. Not found. Similar publication: Adams GA, Feuerstein IA. Platelet adhesion and release: interfacial concentration of released materials. Am J Physiol. 1981;240(1):H99-H108.

Ref. 56. Not found.

Ref. 60. Misspelled, wrong bibliographic description. Correct: Babitch J. Channel hands. Nature. 1990;346(6282):321-322.

Ref. 61. Misspelled, wrong bibliographic description. Correct: Bennett CF, Balcarek JM, Varrichio A, Crooke ST. Molecular cloning and complete amino-acid sequence of form-I phosphoinositide-specific phospholipase C. Nature. 1988;334(6179):268-270.

Ref. 66. Not found.

Ref. 75. Not found. Remotely similar: Conklin BR, Chabre O, Wong YH, Federman AD, Bourne HR. Recombinant Gq alpha. Mutational activation and coupling to receptors and phospholipase C. J Biol Chem. 1992;267(1):31-34.

Ref. 81. Not found.

Ref. 94. Not found. Remotely similar: Eastell R. Forearm fracture. Bone. 1996;18(3 Suppl):203S-207S.

Ref. 100. Not found.

Ref. 105. Not found.

Ref. 130. Not found.

Ref. 151. Not found.

Ref. 163. Not found.

Ref. 169. Not found.

Ref. 170. Not found.

Ref. 172. Not found.

Ref. 177. Not found. Remotely similar: Tilly BC, van Paridon PA, Verlaan I, Wirtz KW, de Laat SW, Moolenaar WH. Inositol phosphate metabolism in bradykinin-stimulated human A431 carcinoma cells. Relationship to calcium signalling. Biochem J. 1987;244(1):129-135.

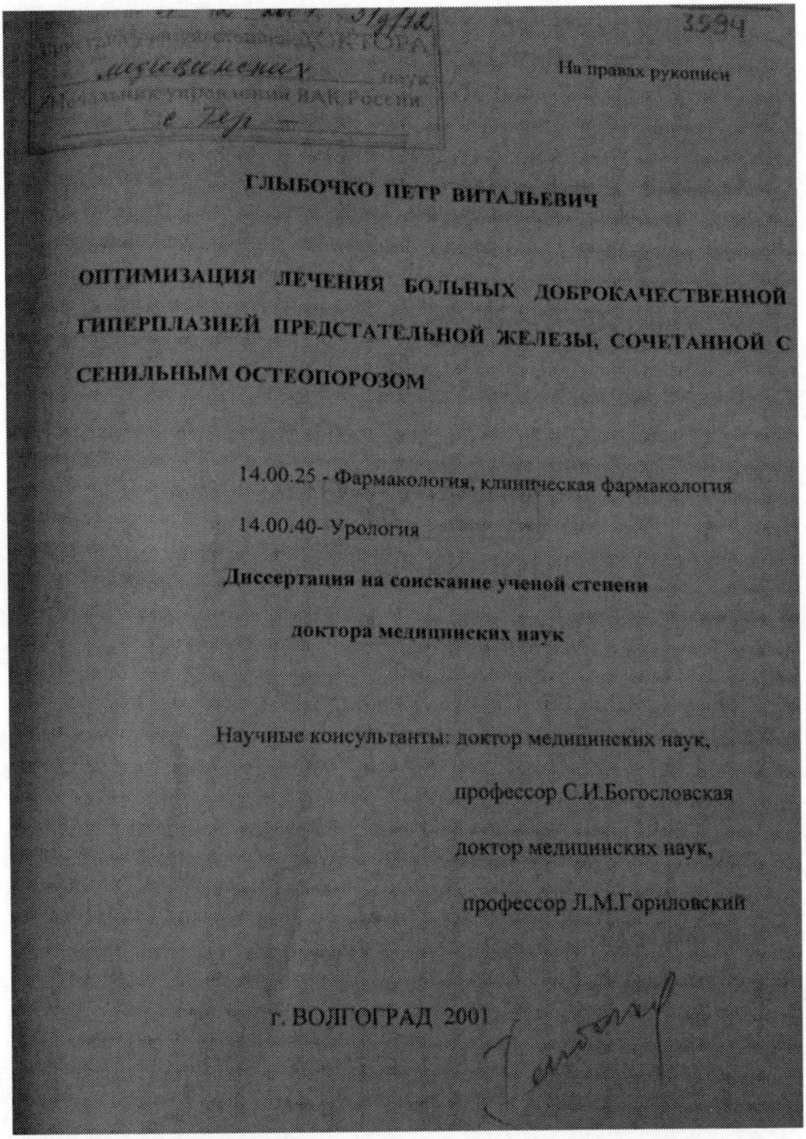

На правах рукописи

ГЛЫБОЧКО ПЕТР ВИТАЛЬЕВИЧ

ОПТИМИЗАЦИЯ ЛЕЧЕНИЯ БОЛЬНЫХ ДОБРОКАЧЕСТВЕННОЙ ГИПЕРПЛАЗИЕЙ ПРЕДСТАТЕЛЬНОЙ ЖЕЛЕЗЫ, СОЧЕТАННОЙ С СЕНИЛЬНЫМ ОСТЕОПОРОЗОМ

14.00.25 - Фармакология, клиническая фармакология

14.00.40- Урология

Диссертация на соискание ученой степени

доктора медицинских наук

Научные консультанты: доктор медицинских наук,

профессор С.И.Богословская

доктор медицинских наук,

профессор Л.М.Гориловский

г. ВОЛГОГРАД 2001

Figure 1.2. The title page of the doctoral thesis (dissertation) of the chancellor of the First Moscow Medical University (previously named I.M. Sechenov Medical Academy) Piotr Glybochko [22].

5

установлено, что увеличение метаболизма андрогенов приводит к гиперплазии предстательной железы (Питель Ю.А. с соавт., 1994).

Перестройка гормональной регуляции в процессе старения организма также приводит к поражению опорно-двигательного аппарата и развитию сенильного остеопороза (Price C., 1993), в основе которого лежит изменение эстрогенового баланса и нарушение чувствительности гормональных рецепторов (Петров В.И. с соавт., 2000).

При старении организма усиливающиеся резорбтивные процессы в костной ткани и гиперпластические в предстательной железе нередко обусловливают сочетанное развитие остеопороза и ДГП.

Данные о сочетанной патологии пожилого возраста предстательной железы и костной ткани достаточно скудны. Так в работах E.Krall с соавторами (1995;1998) указывается, что распространенность остеопенического синдрома у больных доброкачественной гиперплазией простаты составляет 42%.

В списке лит-ры другой год.

Несмотря на поражение различных систем: опорно-двигательного аппарата и предстательной железы эти заболевания имеют ряд общих патогенетических звеньев, и воздействие эффективного и безопасного комбинированного лечения при этом будет благоприятно влиять не только на клиническое течение ДГП и остеопороза, но и способствовать повышению качества жизни.

15

затруднить своевременную диагностику рака предстательной железы. При оценке результатов исследования ПСА у пациентов, длительно принимающих финастерид, следует учитывать, что и показатели ПСА в этой группе в 2 раза ниже по сравнению с соответствующей возрастной нормой. Также установлено, что на фоне терапии финастеридом свободный и общий ПСА уменьшаются в равной степени, в то время как при раке предстательной железы их соотношение практически не изменяется и может быть использовано в качестве диагностического критерия (Wojno K.J., Beduschi M.C., England B.E. et al., 1997).Уродинамическими исследованиями продемонстрировано объективное уменьшение признаков инфравезикальной обструкции на фоне снижения внутрипузырного давления во время мочеиспускания при лечении финастеридом (Keetch D.W, 1997). Финастерид хорошо переносится больными. Наиболее значимые побочные реакции: импотенция - 3,7%, снижение либидо - 3,3%, уменьшение объема эякулята - 2,6% (Stoner E., 1992). Однако через 4 года наблюдения уменьшается число пациентов, предъявлявших жалобы на половые расстройства, а значения указанных показателей снижаются до 2,1; 1,5 и 0,3% соответственно.

Обобщенные данные большинства исследований свидетельствуют о том, что клинически значимое улучшение и уменьшение объема предстательной железы наступают примерно у 30% больных, причем у

Figure 1.3. (Continued).

ДГП, приводит к повышению тонуса гладкомышечных структур основания мочевого пузыря, задней уретры и предстательной железы. Этот механизм, по мнению большинства исследователей, ответствен за развитие динамической обструкции при ДГП (Cine M., 1986).

Эффект α-АБ зависит от избирательности действия на различные подтипы рецепторов. Установлена преимущественная роль α1-АР в патогенезе ДГП (Caine M. et al., 1975; Shapiro E., 1992; Chapple C.R. et al., 1989). В нашей стране одна из первых публикаций по этой теме принадлежит Ю.А. Пытелю и соавт (1988).

Дальнейшая идентификация α1-АР, присутствующих в различных тканях, с помощью фармакологических и молекулярно-биологических методов выявила 3 подтипа рецепторов: α1A, α1B, α1D. Серией исследований было установлено, что подтип α1A в основном присутствует в предстательной железе человека и составляет до 70% всех ее α1-АР (Schalken J.A et al., 1994). Считается, что этот подтип преимущественно ответственен за сокращение гладкомышечных элементов железы и в наибольшей степени влияет на развитие динамической обструкции при ДГП (Miranda H.F. et al., 1994). Назначение α-АБ приводит к снижению тонуса гладкомышечных структур шейки мочевого пузыря и предстательной железы, что в свою очередь проявляется уменьшением уретрального сопротивления и как следствие - уменьшение инфравезикальной обструкции.

215

55.Arams A., Fenrstein J. Platelet adhesion and release// Amer. J. Physiol.-1999.-V.240.-P.34-39.

56.Atkinson A., Anc D., Putney P. Nature of the receptor-regulated calcium pool// Cell.-1992.-V.2.-P.45-49.

57.Avdonin P., Cheglakov I., Mazaev A. Evidence for the receptor-operated cflcium channel// Thromb.Res.-1987.-V.47.-P.21-23.

58.Asch A., Bamwell R. Isolation of thrombospondin receptor// J.Clin.Invest.-1993.-V.79.-P.56-59.

59.Ault K., Tilslan C. Reactions of normal cell to enzymes // PNAS.-1983.-V.56.-P.309-312.

60.Babich J. Channel hands// Nature.-1993.-V.346.-P.89-93.

61.Bennet C., Balcerek J., Crooke S. Molecular cloning// Nature.-1988.-V.334.-P.268-271.

62.Aragona C., Sagiv P., Ambur N. Balance of prolactin in BPH. /Urology. -1978.- №3. - P.25-29.

63.Barry M., Lucas F. Steroides hormones in aging moles.// Y. Endocrin Res.-1998.-P.114-117.

64.Barrett-Connor E. The economic α human cost of osteoporotic fracture./ Amer.Y.Med. - 1995.- №98 (2_A). - P.35-44

65.Bikle D. Pathogenesis of vertebral crush../ Age Aging.- 1997.-№3. - P.72-77.

66.Bouton M., Sandgren M., Riggs B. Sensation of gteroides receptors./ YAMA. - 1997.- №5.- P.27-29.

Figure 1.3. (Continued).

216

67.Breyer C., Black S., Caplan R. The hemodynamic speed in BPH.// Sonooce. - 1997.- №2. - P.36-41.

68.Chong B., Yong L. Focus on NMDA receptors// Sci.-1994.-P.204-207.

69.Chingard M., Loventry S., Petrin K. Distmet neuronal forms of phosphorylation// Proc. Nat. Acad. Sci. US.-1994.-V.175.-P.15-24.

70.Chait V., Chong S.// Sci.-1980.- P.23-27.

71.Chen A., Leunf S. Studies of the mechanism of action of a new antagonist cell reactions// J. Pharmacol.-1995.-V.51.-P.151-159.

72.Chien W., Mohal R., Clusin W. Effect of thrombin on calcium homeostasis// J. Clin. Invest.-1991.-V.85.- P.1436-1443.

73.Clemetson R., Charbe O., Wong Y. Recombinant G// J.Biol.Chem.-1995.- V.267.-P.31-34.

74.Coller A., waslam r., Hurt D. Binding G-subunits phosphoguesterase// Biochem.J.-1995.-V.276.

75.Conkin B., Federman A., Bourne H.// J.Chem.-1992.-V.87.-P.67-69.

76.Codiņa J., Bohen S. The fluxes ion channels// Sci.-1989.-V.239.-P.1191-1193.

77.Connoly R., Yarg L. Excitatory acids// Biochem.J.-1995.-V.251.-P.15-19.

78.Conrad D., Chabre Y. Types channels cell// Biochem.J.-1991.-V.259.-P.931-933.

79.Colman P. Evidence for a role of rapl proteins in cells// Cell.-1983.- V.267.-P.334-339.

217

80.Crock M. Mammalian phospholipase C// Cell Calcium.-1991.-V.10.-P.309-313.

81.Craro E., Person S., Masater S. Effects of biologics// Cell.-1996.-V.34.-P.67-69.

82.Cooper C., Campion G., Melton L. Hip fracture in the eldery.// Osteoporosis. Int.- 1992. - №4. - P.646-650.

83.Cohen C. Proteins of erythrocytes membrane./Cell. - 1992. -№12 (5). - P.56-59.

84.Cagh Y., Nojima S. Hormonal balanse in BPH./ Y. Endocr. Res.- 1992.-№19.- P.74-78.

85.Cutolo M., Paolo N., Noric S. Semle osteoporosis./ Y. Bone Mineral. Res.-1998.- №12.- P.39-44.

86.Daniell H. The regulation of prostatic growth. In: Proceedings on BPH Monaco.- 1993.- P.75-115.

87.Delmas P., Peterson L. Growth factors in aging males./ Y. Endocrin.- 1996.-№5.- P:13.

88.Denis L., Cooper C., Williams R. Management of prostate. // Urol. Clin.-1998.-№23.- P. 87-97.

89.Dochec T., Common S., Korban R. Components of cells membrane.// Cell.-1994.- №62. - P.56-59.

90.Dreher K. Blood rheology in BPH. //Blood Res. - 1990.-V.37.-P.201-207.

91.Farid N., Noderman P. Development of immunity in BPH.// Y. Clin. Res.-1990.- №19.- P.234-237.

Figure 1.3. (Continued).

218

92.Frea B., Brownez W., Nevit M. Releasing factors in BPH./ Am. Y. Med.- 1997.-№16. - P.977-983.

93.Edkins L., Gardsell P. The predictive volue osteoclastes./ Calc. Tissue.- 1995.- №12.- P.90-94.

94.Eastell R. Epidemiology of fractures. / Osteoporosis. - 1990.- №1. - P.33-35.

95.Ehrly A., Malkov P., Peterson L. Deformobility of erythaocytes.// Hocmotel. - 1976.- №3.- P.32-37.

96.Elomaa I., Petricaa P., Penter S. Elderly pationts with arthritis / Y. Bone mineral Res.- 1992.- №22.- P.3-7.

97.Eriksen E., Plow P., Havigen N. Bone density α fractures/ Y. Bone Miner. Res.- 1998. - №2.- P.7A.

98.Evans A., Marel G., Lancaster E. Bone moss is low in relatives of osteoporotic patients.// Ann. Intern. Med.- 1998. - №106. - P.870-875.

99.Gambee J., Actories K., Jakobs K. Evidence for two GTPase activated by thrombin // Biochem J.- 1990. - V.237. - P.669-674.

100.Garcia J. Mechanism of ion permeation // Nature. - 1994.- V.45.- P.89-93.

101.Gasper N., Beridge M., Aspley S. Pharmacological modulation of blowly PML // Biochem J. - 1993. - V.249. - P.883-889.

102.Gale R., Chueh S., Reynolds G. An intracellular Ca-dependent pump in PML // Nature. - 1993. - V.56. - P.289-294.

103.Gend A., Choi W., Suh P. Phospholinase C I u II isozymes // PNAS. - 1990. - V.65.

219

104.Ginsberg R. Adhesion platelets: molecular properties // J. Biol. Chem. - 1995. - V.267. - P.28-51.

105.Glenn G., Helzwerth J. Receptors activate mobilization Ca // PNAS. - 1989.- V.87.

106.Goorge J., Ueda T., Noel M. Calcium release from endoplasmic reticulum by a guanine nucleotide // Nature. - 1990. - V.320. - P. 461-464.

107.Goldyne M., Striessnig J. Molecular properties of membrane channels // Rev. Physiol. - 1989. - V.114. - P.1-17.

108.Golgen A., Rogan C., Raid G. The purification of myo-inositol // Biochem J. - 1999. - V.13. - P. 301-307.

109.Glomset J. Epidermal growth factor // J. Bioch. - 1976.- V.34.- P.89-91.

110.Gregory J. Cation gradient of thrombin // J.Biohem. - 1989. - V.327. - P.12-19.

111.Grem P., Fong H., Ocken K. Proteins control diverse pathways of transmembrane signaling // FASEB. - 1995.- V.3. - P.215-224.

112.Gramse L., Rosenthal W. Angiotensin II - induced stimulation of cell // EMBO. - 1990. - V. 7. - P.619-624.

113.Green S. Atriopeptin II decreases free Ca // J. Phy. 1989. - V.251.- P.789-794.

114.Gremse L., Bolla T., Calt C. ITP links to specific receptor and release microsomal subunits // PNAS. - 1987. - V.84. - P.195-199.

115.Grandt R., Jonston D. Noradrenaline and beta-receptor agonists increase activity cells // Nature. - 1993. - V.327. - P.620-625.

Figure 1.3. (Continued).

221

127.Kelly P., Pocock N. Dietary calcium, sex hormones α bone density./ Br. Med. Y.- 1990.- №300. - P.1361-1364.

128.Kledzik G., Markovic V. Prolactin production in old males./ Y. Clin. Res.- 1998.- №6.- P. 215-227

129.Kley H. Metabolism of testosteroids./ Y. Clin. Endocrinal. Metab.- 1995.- №9. - P.15-19.

130.Klover P., Riggs B. Osteoblastic functions./ Bone Miner.- 1991.-№3. - P.215-217.

131.Krall E., Dawson B. Heritage α life style deferminants of bone mineral density./ Y. Bone Miner. Res. - 1993.- №8.- P.1-9.

132.La Celle P., Bally S., Francis K. Erythrocytes as model for distinetion./ Halmotol.- 1987.- №3.- P.301-307.

133.Lahita R. Sexual hormones in BPH./ Y.Urology. - 1992.- №63 (2).- P.341-346.

134.Lorand N. Marshall P.Calcium as modeling ion./ Cell.- 1995.- $№27_A$.- P.39-44.

135.Lotz J., Hosoi T. Associatition of porat-hormone α Vit. D.//Bone.- 1995.- №13.- P.64-68.

136.Looket A., Wakner H. Prevalance of low femoral bone density./ Y.Bone Mineral.- 1995.- №45. - P.101-107.

137.Leviele M., Partin A. Influence of age α endocrine factors in BPH./Y. Clin. Endocrin.- 1995.- №7. - P.123-127.

223

150.Penner R., Matthews G., Neher E. Regulation of calcium influx by second messengers // Nature.- 1988.- V.334. - P.499-504.

151.Perussia B., Mauger Y. Calcium mediaties the inteconversion between two states of the receptor // J. Biol. Chem. - 1990. - V.265.- P.78-85.

152.Petrson P. Role receptor - mediated control in calcium mobilization// Cell Calcium.- 1991. - V.10. -P.375-383.

153.Phillips D., Pipili E. Platelet membrane potentials // Thromb. Res. - 1988. - V.54.- P.645-649.

154.Phueller S., Gaugler B., Metzger H. Isolation of homologous and heterologous complexes between platelet and PML // FEBS.-1989.- V.164.- P.154-160.

155.Pierscherber M. Structural and functional aspects of homeostasis in cells // Eeurop. J. Biochem. - 1993. - V.193. - P.599-622.

156.Plow P. Human cDNA in PML rap1 and rap2 //Oncogene. - 1989.- V.3.- P.201-204.

157.Pol U., Yones R. Thromboxane - induced phosphotidate formation in pleatelets // Biochem. J.- 1988.- V.219.- P.833-842.

158.Pretter C., Weiss S., Haddes R. Model for receptor - regulated calcium entry // Cell Calcium. - 1993. - V.7. - P.1-12.

159.Pytela R., Hess P., Eakes A. Conformational changes associated with ion permeation // Nature.- 1992.-V.333.-P.373-376.

160.Rabson P., Chen M., Digiusto D. Nitrendipine - induced inhibition of PML // Cell Calcium. - 1992.- V.12. - P.313-323.

Figure 1.3. (Continued).

224

161.Rand J., Erne P. Platelet membrane calmodulin - dependent receptor // J. Hypertension.-1998.-V.8.-P.159-166.

162.Rall S. Why are so mane biological systems periodic? // Progr.Neur.-1988.-V.29.

163.Ramachi G. Acetylcholine and cholecystokinin receptors functionally couple to g-protein // FEBS.-1993.-V.23.

164.Rasmussen H., Spincher K. Cyclyc AMP-independent dual regulation // EMBO. - 1990.-V.7. - P.627-634.

165.Renesto A., Feinberg H. ITP - release from PML platelets // Biochem. J. - 1992.-V.150.

166.Resin K., Bruno P. Glutamate- stimulated guanine nucleotide - mediated turnover by cAMP// J. Neurochem. - 1986.- V.78.-P.90-94.

167.Reuter H. Ion channels in cardiac cell membranes// Annu Rev. Physiol.-1987.-V.46.

168.Rink T., Smith S., Hallam T. What turns platelets on? // Trends Biochem.-1987.- V.9.-P.215-219.

169.Snyder S. Sequence similarity of pec //Nature. - 1989.- V.332.-P.56-62.

170.Spilberg R. Purification and characterization of a new isozyme of thiol // J. Biol. Chem.- 1987.-V.90.-P.34-38.

171.Spact G. Binding of inositol by platelets // Biochem. J.- 1976.- V.233.-P.23.

172.Storck Y., Hollger N., Zimberman R. Release of Ca from intracellular store // Nature.- 1995.- V.306.- P.67-69.

225

173.Sternweis P. The purificated alpha subunit of G proteins // J. Biol. Chem.- 1986.- V.251.- P.631-637.

174.Swann K. Thimesosol causes calcium oscillations // FEBS Lett.- 1991.- V.278.- P.175-178.

175.Tokada Y., Katz A. G-protein mediated regulation of ion channels // Annu. Rev. Physiol.- 1989.-V.52.- P.293-305.

176.Tech L., Horie M., Makita T. Synthetic obrial peptide // Nature.- 1990.- V.237.- P.803.

177.Tilly K., Verlean I. Inositol phosphate metabolism to calcium signalling // Biochem. J.- 1990.- V.244.- P.129-135.

178.Tomlinson R. A novel 100 kDc protein localisated to receptor- enrished endosomes // Biochem. J.- 1989.- V.272.- P.453-458.

179.Torti M., Chadwik C., Fleischer S. Phosphorylation states of receptor PML and platelets // Biophys. J. - 1995.- V.266.- P. 235-243.

180.Thelen M., Estevez V., Ferris C. Receptor proteins: isolation and characterization // PNAS.- 1998.- V. 88.- P.3165-3169.

181.Toyshime S., Bollon C. Complite characterization from brain phosphoinositide // J. Biol. Chem.- 1989.- V.236.-P.897-900.

Figure 1.3. Copies from the text and reference list of the thesis [22]. Many authors' names present in the text are absent in the reference list, which is a form of misquoting. Many authors' names are misspelled. Further details are in the text.

References

[1] von Elm E. Research integrity: collaboration and research needed. *Lancet* 2007;370:1403-4.

[2] Vlasov VV. Emerging problems of medical ethics in Russia: medical practice and research. *Kardiologiia* 2002;42(5):81-84.

[3] Gordon AG. Never cite sight unseen. *Am J Obstet Gynecol* 1998;178:627.

[4] Jargin SV. Overestimation of Chernobyl consequences: poorly substantiated information published. *Radiat Environ Biophys* 2020;49:743-5.

[5] Asai A, Okita T, Enzo A. Conflicting messages concerning current strategies against research misconduct in Japan: a call for ethical spontaneity. *J Med Ethics* 2016;42:524-7.

[6] Iargin SV. The message about unreliability of publications. *Klin Khir* 2011;(6):69-70.

[7] Severgina ES, Pal'tsev MA. Hypoplastic dysplasia as one of the forms of nephropathy. *Arkh Patol* 1989;51(10):58-63.

[8] Severgina LO, Gurevich SI. Ultrastructural assessment of the role of dysangiogenesis in congenital hydronephrosis. *Arkh Patol* 2014;76(6):51-55.

[9] Jargin SV. On the endoscopic methods used with questionable indications. *J Surgery* 2016;4:6.

[10] Jargin SV. Invasive procedures with questionable indications. *Ann Med Surg* 2014;3:126-9.

[11] Jargin SV. Some aspects of renal biopsy for research. *Int J Nephrol Kidney Failure* 2015;1:8.

[12] Jargin SV. Pathology in the former Soviet Union: scientific misconduct and related phenomena. *Dermatol Pract Concept* 2011;1:75-81.

[13] Jargin SV. Memoirs, Articles, Documents. *Bloggingbooks,* 2015. ISBN-13:978-3-8417-7193-3.

[14] Smith R. Research misconduct: The poisoning of the well. *J R Soc Med* 2006;99:232-7.

[15] Jargin SV. Scientific Papers and Patents on Substances with Unproven Effects. *Recent Pat Drug Deliv Formul* 2019;13:37-45. Part 2. 160-173.

[16] Babalola O, Grant-Kels JM, Parish LC. Ethical dilemmas in journal publication. *Clin Dermatol* 2012;30:231-6.

[17] Cowell HR. Ethical responsibilities of editors, reviewers, and authors. *Clin Orthop Relat Res* 2000;378:83-89.

[18] Jargin SV. Unfair practices in the publication process on the part of editors. *Molodoi Uchenyi - Young Sci* 2016;(20):34-40.

[19] Jargin SV. Alcohol consumption by Russian workers before and during the economical reforms of the 1990s. *Int J High Risk Behav Addic* 2013;2:48-50.

[20] Jargin SV. Why fortified wines have disappeared. *Vinodelie-i-Vinogradarstvo (Winemaking and viticulture)* 2014;(3):19.

[21] Jargin SV. Development of antiatherosclerotic drugs on the basis of cell models. *Int J Pharmacol Phytochem Ethnomed* 2015;1:10-14.

[22] Glybochko PV. *Treatment optimization of benign prostatic hyperplasia combined with senile osteoporosis.* Doctoral dissertation. Saratov, 2001. (in Russian)

Chapter 2

EXAMPLES OF PLAGIARISM

Before the 1990s, partial isolation from the external world allowed an illusion in the former Soviet Union that plagiarism was a normal scientific activity. Some examples of plagiarism from the recent past are shown here. These examples are only a tip of the iceberg. Among plagiarists are functionaries occupying high positions in academies and universities. Students and young researchers learn from them that scientific misconduct brings success and profit.

Five publications are quoted below: two journal articles, one handbook of pathology, and two textbooks of pathological anatomy (one of them in three volumes). All these books were issued by the Moscow Medical Academy and a leading institution in Saint Petersburg, bear official recommendations of the Ministry of Health, and are widely in use.

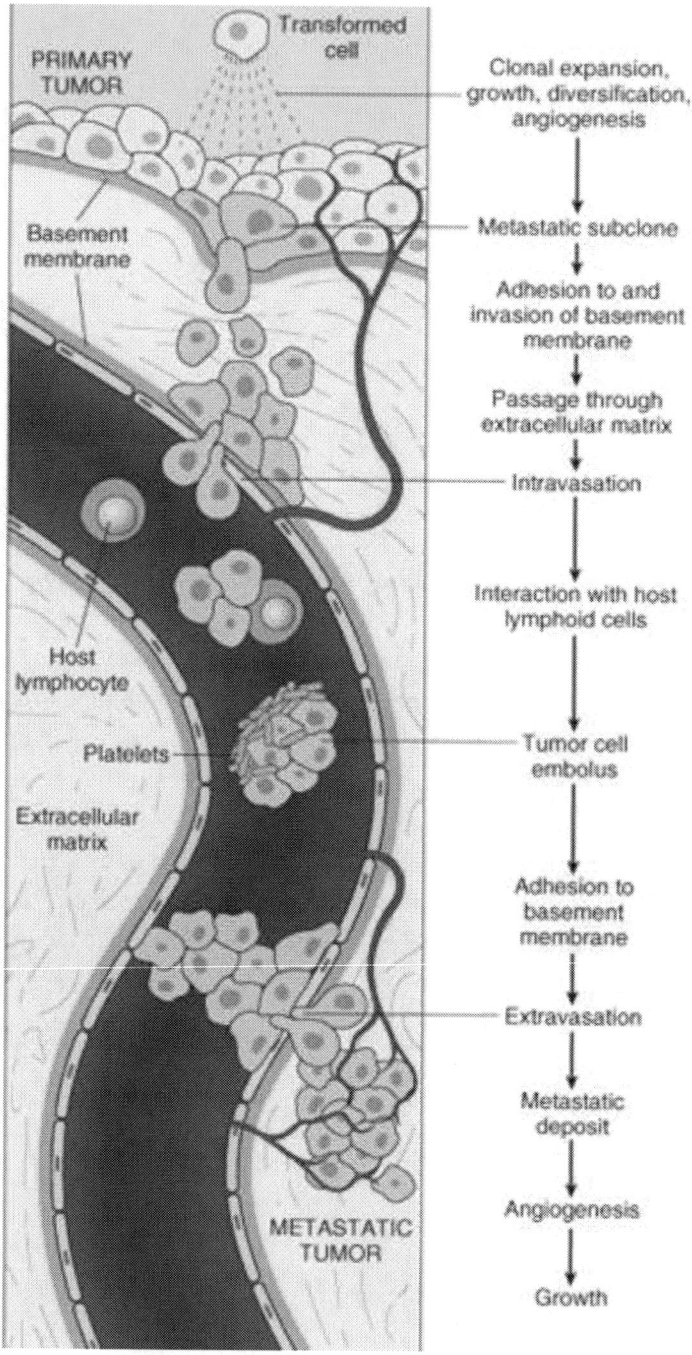
Transformed cell
PRIMARY TUMOR
Clonal expansion, growth, diversification, angiogenesis
Basement membrane
Metastatic subclone
Adhesion to and invasion of basement membrane
Passage through extracellular matrix
Intravasation
Interaction with host lymphoid cells
Host lymphocyte
Tumor cell embolus
Platelets
Extracellular matrix
Adhesion to basement membrane
Extravasation
Metastatic deposit
Angiogenesis
METASTATIC TUMOR
Growth

a)

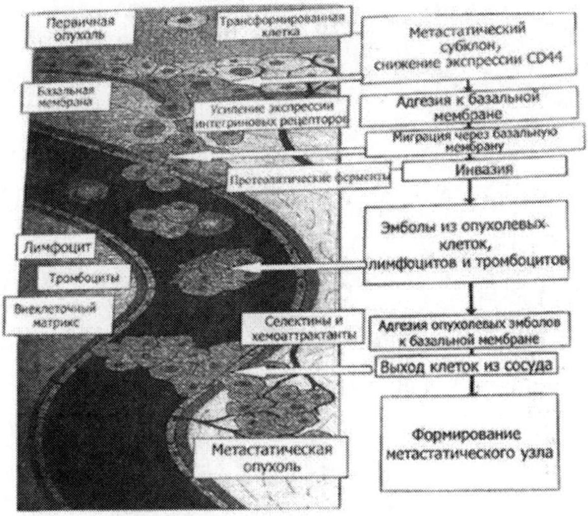

Рис. 3. Участие адгезивных молекул в метастатическом каскаде.

b)

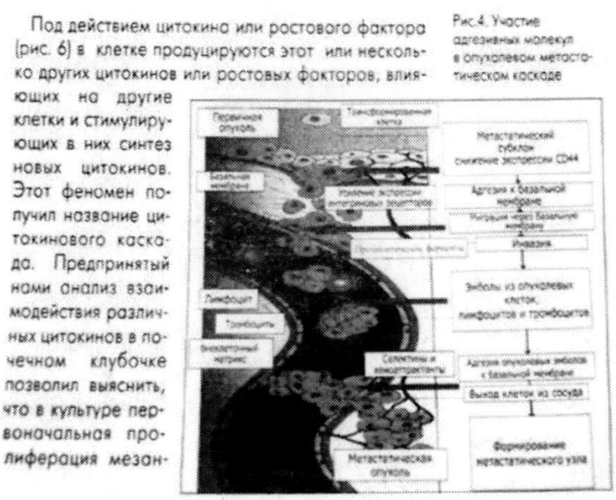

Под действием цитокина или ростового фактора (рис. 6) в клетке продуцируются этот или несколько других цитокинов или ростовых факторов, влияющих на другие клетки и стимулирующих в них синтез новых цитокинов. Этот феномен получил название цитокинового каскада. Предпринятый нами анализ взаимодействия различных цитокинов в почечном клубочке позволил выяснить, что в культуре первоначальная пролиферация мезан-

Рис.4. Участие адгезивных молекул в опухолевом метастатическом каскаде

c)

Figure 2.1a-c. A diagram that appeared in the textbook by R.S. Cotran, V. Kumar, and S.L. Robbins, Robbins' Pathologic Basis of Disease (Philadelphia: W.B. Saunders Co., 1994) on page 277 [1] has been reproduced in two articles without references to the source. Figure 2.1b shows the diagram in an article that appeared in the Journal of the Russian Academy of Medical Science [2]. Most of the inscriptions on the diagram are translated literally. Figure 2.1c shows the same diagram in the journal Vrach (The Physician) [3].

Table 8-1. CLASSES OF HUMAN ENDOPARASITES AND THEIR HABITATS

TAXONOMIC CLASS	SIZE	SITE OF PROPAGATION	SAMPLE SPECIES AND ITS DISEASE	
Viruses	20–30 nm	Obligate intracellular	Poliovirus	Poliomyelitis
Chlamydiae	200–1000 nm	Obligate intracellular	*C. trachomatis*	Trachoma
Rickettsiae	300–1200 nm	Obligate intracellular	*R. prowazekii*	Typhus fever
Mycoplasmas	125–350 nm	Extracellular	*M. pneumoniae*	Atypical pneumonia
Bacteria, spirochetes, mycobacteria	0.8–15 μm	Cutaneous Mucosal Extracellular Facultative intracellular	*Staphylococcus epidermidis* *Vibrio cholerae* *Streptococcus pneumoniae* *M. tuberculosis*	Wound infection Cholera Pneumonia Tuberculosis
Fungi imperfecti	2–200 μm	Cutaneous Mucosal Extracellular Facultative intracellular	*Trichophyton* sp. *Candida albicans* *Sporothrix schenkii* *Histoplasma capsulatum*	Tinea pedis (athlete's foot) Thrush Sporotrichosis Histoplasmosis
Protozoa	1–50 mm	Mucosal Extracellular Facultative intracellular Obligate intracellular	*G. lamblia* *Trypanosoma gambiense* *Trypanosoma cruzi* *L. donovani*	Giardiosis Sleeping sickness Chagas' disease Kala-azar
Helminths	3 mm–10 m	Mucosal Extracellular Intracellular	*Enterobius vermicularis* *Wuchereria bancrofti* *Trichinella spiralis*	Oxyuriasis Filariasis Trichinosis

a)

Таблица 14.1. **Эндопаразиты человека**

Таксономический класс	Размер возбудителей	Вид и место паразитирования	Названия некоторых основных возбудителей из указанных таксономических классов	Вызываемые заболевания
Вирусы	20—30 нм	Облигатные внутриклеточные паразиты	Вирус полиомиелита (полиовирус)	Полиомиелит
Хламидии	200—1000 нм	То же	Chlamydia trachomatis	Трахома
Риккетсии	300—1200 нм	» »	Rickettsia prowazekii	Сыпной тиф
Микоплазмы	125—350 нм	Внеклеточные паразиты	Mycoplasma pneumoniae	Атипичная пневмония
Бактерии, спирохеты, микобактерии	0,8—15 мкм	Паразитируют в коже, слизистых оболочках; являются внеклеточными и факультативными внутриклеточными паразитами	Staphylococcus epidermidis Vibrio cholerae Streptococcus pneumoniae Mycobacterium tuberculosis	Раневые инфекции Холера Пневмония Туберкулез
Грибы несовершенные	2—200 мкм	То же	Группа грибов Trichophyton Candida albicans Sporothrix schenkii Histoplasma capsulatum	Эпидермофития стопы Кандидоз Споротрихоз Гистоплазмоз
Простейшие	1—50 мм	Паразитируют в слизистых оболочках в качестве факультативных и облигатных внутриклеточных паразитов	Giardia lamblia Trypanosoma gambiense Trypanosoma cruzi Leishmania donovani	Лямблиоз Сонная болезнь Болезнь Шагаса (C.Chagas) Висцеральный лейшманиоз (кала-азар)
Гельминты	3 мм—10 м	Паразитируют вне и внутри клеток в слизистых оболочках	Enterobius vermicularis Wuchereria bancrofti Trichinella spiralis	Энтеробиоз (оксиуроз) Филяриоз Трихинеллез

b)

Figure 2.2a,b. A table that appeared in Robbins' Pathologic Basis of Disease on page 307 [1] has been reproduced in the textbook Pathologicheskaya Anatomia, by M.A. Paltsev and N.M. Anichkov, printed by the publishing house Meditsina in Moscow in 2001. On page 254 of volume 2 of this work [4], the table can be identified also without knowledge of Russian language because numerals and Latin terms are the same as in the original source.

Table 8–7. SEXUALLY TRANSMITTED INFECTIOUS DISEASES

A. Exclusively or regularly transmitted by sexual contact	
CAUSAL AGENT	**DISEASE MANIFESTATIONS**
Viral	
HIV-I, HIV-II	Acquired immunodeficiency syndrome
Herpesvirus 1, 2 (HSV-1, 2)	Herpes lesions
Papillomaviruses	Condyloma acuminatum, cervical dysplasia, neoplasia
Chlamydial, Mycoplasmal	
Chlamydia trachomatis (L type)	*Lymphogranuloma venereum*
C. trachomatis	Nongonorrheal urethritis, cervicitis
Ureaplasma urealyticum	Nongonorrheal urethritis, cervicitis
Bacterial	
Neisseria gonorrhoeae	Gonorrhea
Treponema pallidum	Syphilis (lues venerea)
Haemophilus ducreyi	Chancroid
Calymmatobacterium donovani	Granuloma inguinale
Protozoal	
Trichomonas vaginalis	Trichomoniasis
By Arthropod	
Phthirus pubis	Pediculosis pubis (crabs)

B. Transmissible sexually or by other means

Viral
Cytomegalovirus, hepatitis B virus, Epstein-Barr virus, molluscum contagiosum virus

Bacterial
Group B streptococci; gram-negative bacilli

Fungal
Candida

Protozoal
Entamoeba histolytica

a)

Figure 2.3a,b. (Continued).

Таблица 14.2. **Инфекции, передающиеся половым путем (венерические болезни)**

Агенты	Заболевания
Венерические заболевания, регулярно передающиеся половым путем	
Вирусы	
HIV-I, HIV-II	Синдром приобретенного иммунодефицита
Вирусы герпеса 1, 2 (HSV-1, -2)	Герпес
Вирусы папилломы (см. рис.14.21)	Остроконечная кондилома, дисплазия эпителия шейки матки, опухоли (см. рис. 14.21)
Хламидии, микоплазмы	
Chlamydia trachomatis (типы L_1, L_2 и L_3)	Паховый лимфогранулематоз
Chlamydia trachomatis (см. табл.14.3)	Негонорейные уретриты и цервициты
Ureaplasma urealyticum	Негонорейные уретриты и цервициты
Бактерии	
Гонококк (Neisseria gonorrhoeae)	Гонорея
Бледная спирохета (Treponema pallidum)	Сифилис (люэс)
Haemophilus ducreyi	Мягкий шанкр (4-я венерическая болезнь)
Calymmatobacterium donovani	Венерическая гранулема (5-я венерическая болезнь)
Влагалищная гарднерелла (G.vaginalis)	Вагинит, цервицит
Простейшие	
Влагалищная трихомонада (T.vaginalis)	Трихомоноз
Членистоногие эктопаразиты	
Лобковая вошь (Phthirus pubis)	Лобковый педикулез
Инфекции, передающиеся половым путем и иными способами	
Вирусы	
Цитомегаловирус, вирус гепатита B, вирус Эпштейна—Барр, вирус контагиозного моллюска	
Бактерии	
Стрептококки группы B, грамотрицательные микробы	
Грибы	
Кандида	
Простейшие	
Амеба (Entamoeba histolytica)	

b)

Figure 2.3a,b. Another table that was published originally in Robbins' Pathologic Basis of Disease on page 340 [1] was reproduced without proper reference in the textbook by M.A. Paltsev and N.M. Anichkov on page 325 [4]. Again, the Latin terms and proper names are recognizable.

HYPOXIA. Hypoxia, an extremely important and common cause of cell injury and cell death, impinges on aerobic oxidative respiration. Loss of blood supply *(ischemia)*, which occurs when arterial flow is impeded by arteriosclerosis or by thrombi, is the most common cause of hypoxia. Another cause is inadequate oxygenation of the blood due to cardiorespiratory failure. Loss of the oxygen-carrying *capacity* of the blood, as in anemia or carbon monoxide poisoning (producing a stable carbon monoxyhemoglobin that blocks oxygen carriage), is a third, less frequent basis of oxygen deprivation. Depending on the severity of the hypoxic state, cells may adapt, undergo injury, or die. For example, if the femoral artery is narrowed, the skeletal muscle cells of the leg may shrink in size (atrophy). This reduction in cell mass achieves a balance between metabolic needs and the available oxygen supply. More severe hypoxia induces injury and cell death.

PHYSICAL AGENTS. Physical agents include mechanical trauma, extremes of temperature (burns and deep cold), sudden changes in atmospheric pressure, radiation, and electric shock (see Chapter 9, Environmental and Nutritional Diseases).

CHEMICAL AGENTS AND DRUGS. The list of chemicals that may produce cell injury defies compilation. Simple chemicals such as glucose or salt in hypertonic concentrations may cause cell injury directly or by deranging electrolyte homeostasis of cells. Even oxygen, in high concentrations, is severely toxic. Trace amounts of agents known as *poisons*, such as arsenic, cyanide, or mercuric salts, may destroy sufficient numbers of cells within minutes to hours to cause death. Other substances, however, are our daily companions: environmental and air pollutants, insecticides, and herbicides; industrial and occupational hazards, such as carbon monoxide and asbestos; social stimuli, such as alcohol and narcotic drugs; and the ever-increasing variety of therapeutic drugs.

a)

ПРИЧИНЫ ПОВРЕЖДЕНИЯ КЛЕТОК

Различают следующие причины повреждения клеток.

1. Гипоксия. Она является исключительно важной и распространенной причиной повреждения и смерти клеток. Уменьшение кровотока (ишемия), возникающее при появлении препятствий в артериях, обычно при атеросклерозе или тромбозе, является основной причиной гипоксии. Другой причиной может быть неадекватная оксигенация крови при сердечно-сосудистой недостаточности. Снижение способности крови к транспортировке кислорода, например при анемии и отравлении CO_2 — третья и наиболее редкая причина гипоксии. В зависимости от тяжести гипоксии клетки могут адаптироваться к ней, повреждаться или погибать.

2. Физические агенты. К ним относят механическую травму, чрезмерное снижение или повышение температуры окружающей среды, внезапные колебания атмосферного давления, радиацию и электрический шок.

3. Химические агенты и лекарства. Даже простые химические соединения, такие как глюкоза и поваренная соль, в повышенных

19 b)

Figure 2.4a,b. The paragraphs about hypoxia, physical agents, chemical agents, and drugs from [1] are reproduced verbatim in the textbook [5]. A mistranslation can be seen, namely, carbon monoxide mistranslated as CO_2.

1. *A normal endogenous substance is produced at a normal or increased rate, but the rate of metabolism is inadequate to remove it.* An example of this type of process is *fatty change* in the liver due to intracellular accumulation of triglycerides.

2. *A normal or abnormal endogenous substance accumulates because it cannot be metabolized or is deposited intracellularly in an amorphous or filamentous form.* One important cause is a genetic enzymatic defect in a specific metabolic pathway, so that some particular metabolite cannot be used. The resulting diseases are referred to as *storage diseases* (discussed in Chapter 5).

3. *An abnormal exogenous substance is deposited* and accumulates because the cell has neither the enzymic machinery to degrade the substance nor the ability to transport it to other sites. Accumulations of carbon particles and such nonmetabolizable chemicals as silica particles are examples of this type of alteration. Viral inclusions also fall into this category and are discussed in Chapter 8.

a)

- во-первых, нормальные эндогенные вещества, которые образуются в нормальном или ускоренном ритме, а скорость метаболизма неадекватна для их удаления. Например, жировые изменения печени, обусловленные внутриклеточным накоплением триглицеридов;
- во-вторых, нормальное или ненормальное накопление эндогенных веществ, которые не могут метаболизироваться. Они откладываются внутри клетки в виде аморфных или филаментозных скоплений. Важной причиной этого является генетический дефект фермента. В результате некоторые продукты метаболизма не могут быть использованы клеткой и развиваются болезни накопления;
- в-третьих, аномальные экзогенные продукты откладываются и аккумулируются, так как клетка не может ни разрушить их с помощью ферментов, ни транспортировать их в другое место. Примерами такого типа повреждений клеток служат отложения частиц угля, кремнезема, а также вирусные включения.

b)

Figure 2.5a,b. The text also taken from Robbins' Pathologic Basis of Disease, page 24 [1] appeared in the textbook titled Rukovodstvo po Obshchei Patologii Cheloveka (Handbook of Human General Pathology), edited by N.K. Khitrov, D.S. Sarkisov, and M.A. Paltsev [6].

References

[1] Cotran RS, Kumar V, Robbins SL. *Robbins' Pathologic Basis of Disease.* Philadelphia: W.B. Saunders Co., 1994.

[2] Pal'tsev MA. [Current approaches to studying the pathogenesis of diseases]. *Vestn Ross Akad Med Nauk* 1999;(9):22-5.

[3] Pal'tsev MA. [Molecular pathology]. Vrach 1999;(6):13.

[4] Paltsev MA, Anichkov NM. *Patologicheskaya Anatomia* [*Pathological anatomy*] Moscow: Medicina, 2001.

[5] Serov VV, Paltsev MA, *Patologicheskaya Anatomia.* Kurs lektsii [*Pathological anatomy. Lectures*] Moscow: Medicina, 1998.

[6] Khitrov NK, Sarkisov D.S., Paltsev MA. *Rukovodstvo po Obshei Patologii Cheloveka* [*Handbook of Human General Pathology*]. Moscow: Meditsina, 1999.

Chapter 3

PLAGIARISM IN DERMATOPATHOLOGY

Further examples are from the field of dermatopathology. The source of the borrowings was the well known Histopathology of the Skin by W.F. Lever and G. Schaumburg-Lever, published by Lippincott in 1975 [1]. The "text borrowings" were found in a textbook edited by G.M. Tsvetkova and V.N. Mordovtsev titled Patomorfologicheskaya diagnostika zabolevanii kozhi (Pathomorphologic Diagnosis of Skin Diseases) [2].

Example 1

The paragraph on Darier's disease is an example of a section translated almost entirely verbatim, with omission of some phrases and words. No reference is made to the original source and no quotation marks are used.

The paragraphs from Lever's Histopathology of the Skin read as follows (p. 72):

> "Histopathology. The characteristic changes of Darier's disease are (1) a peculiar form of dyskeratosis resulting in the formation of corps ronds and grains, (2) suprabasal acantholysis leading to the formation of suprabasal clefts and lacunae, and (3) irregular upward proliferation into the lacunae of papillae lined with a single layer of basal cells, so-called

villi. There are also papillomatosis, acanthosis and hyperkeratosis. The dermis shows a chronic inflammatory infiltrate. In some cases there is downward proliferation of epidermal cells into the dermis.

The corps ronds occur in the upper stratum malpighii, particularly in the granular and horny layers; grains are found in the horny layer and as acantholytic cells within the lacunae. Corps ronds possess a central large, round, homogenous, basophilic mass that is surrounded by clear halo. In virtue of their size and conspicuous halo corps ronds stand out clearly. The central basophilic mass consists either of the pycnotic nucleus or of dyskeratotic material or both. Peripheral to the halo lies additional basophilic dyskeratotic material as a shell. The nonstaining halo may be partially replaced by homogenous, eosinophilic dyskeratotic material. In contrast to the corps ronds, the grains are much less conspicuous. They resemble parakeratotic cells ...” [1].

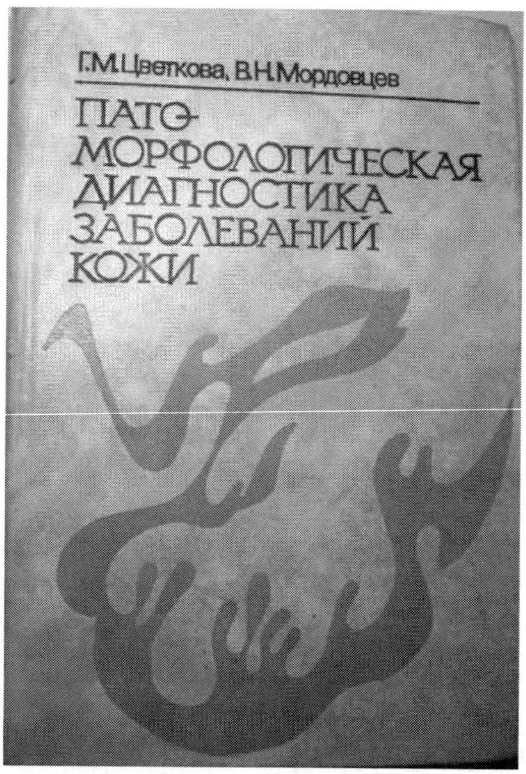

Figure 3.1. The cover of the textbook by G.M. Tsvetkova and V.N. Mordovtsev [2].

The text continues on page 73 as follows:

> "In hypertrophic lesions of Darier's disease one occasionally can observe considerable downward proliferation of the epidermis, either as a proliferation of basal cells or as pseudocarcinomatous hyperplasia. The proliferations of basal cells consist of long, narrow cords composed of two rows of basal cells separated by narrow lacunar spacce (Beerman; Krinitz). The vesicles, which occur in rare instances ..." [1].

The corresponding paragraphs in the Russian textbook on page 89 (Figure 3.2) can be translated verbatim as follows:

> "Histopathology. The characteristic histologic signs of Darier's disease are a peculiar form of dyskeratosis with formation of corps ronds and grains, suprabasal acantholysis leading to the formation of lacunae, irregular proliferation in the lacunae of papillae lined with a single layer of basal cells, so-called villi There are also papillomatosis, acanthosis and hyperkeratosis, and in the dermis - a chronic inflammatory infiltrate" [2]. Note: The word "villi" has an equivalent in Russian: "vorsiny;" but the plagiarists transliterated the "villi" in Cyrillic letters.
>
> "The corps ronds occur in the upper stratum malpighii, particularly in the granular and horny layers; grains are found in the horny layer and as acantholytic cells within the lacunae. Corps ronds possess a central large, round, homogenous, basophilic mass that is surrounded by clear halo. In the peripheral part of a corp rond (outside halo) lies additional basophilic dyskeratotic material as a shell [The translation of this sentence differs slightly from the original, and the sense is altered]. The non-staining halo may be partially replaced by eosinophilic dyskeratotic material... . In contrast to the corps ronds, the grains are much less conspicuous. They resemble parakeratotic cells... . In hypertrophic lesions one can observe considerable proliferation of the epidermis, as pseudocarcinomatous hyperplasia or appearance of narrow outgrowths composed of several rows of basal cells separated by narrow space or lacunas. The vesicles occur sometimes in the epidermis..." [2].

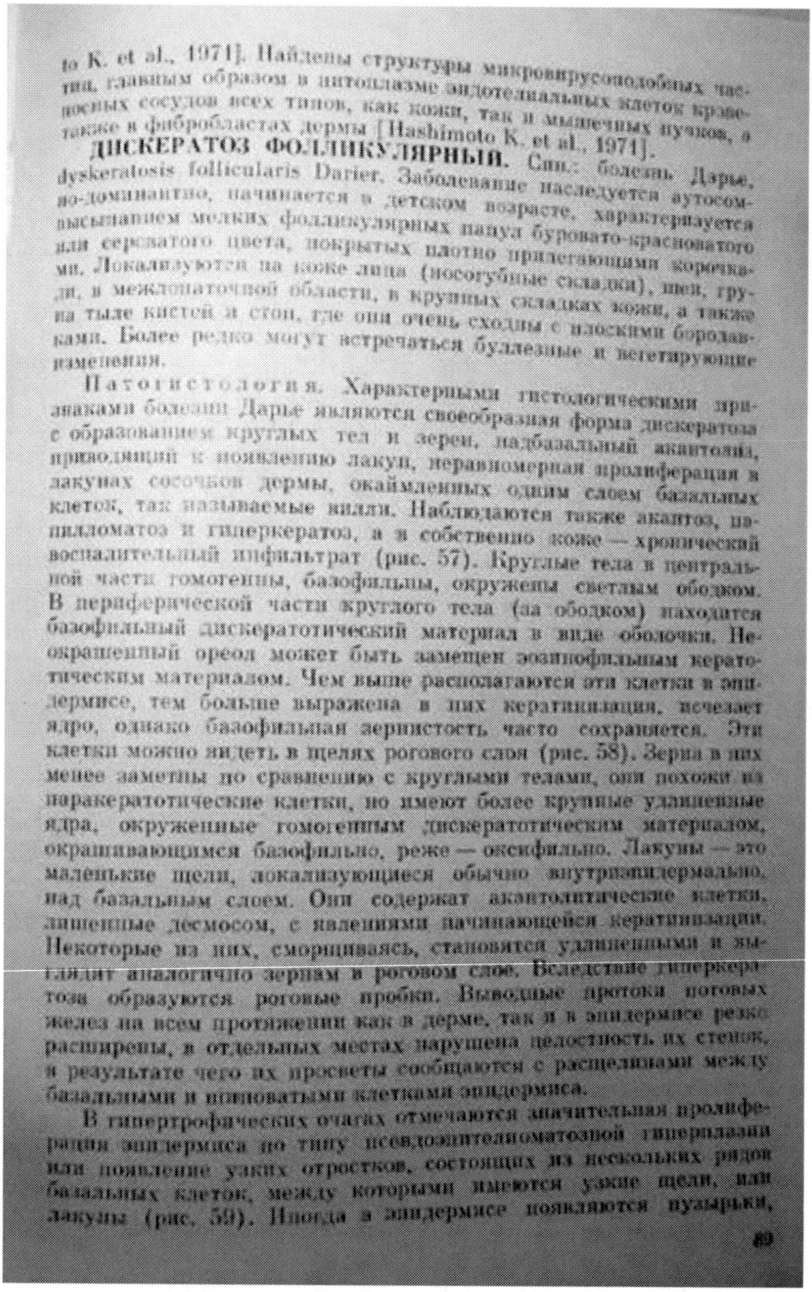

to K. et al., 1971]. Найдены структуры микровирусоподобных час тиц, главным образом в цитоплазме эндотелиальных клеток крове носных сосудов всех типов, как кожи, так и мышечных пучков, а также в фибробластах дермы [Hashimoto K. et al., 1971].

ДИСКЕРАТОЗ ФОЛЛИКУЛЯРНЫЙ. Син.: болезнь Дарье, dyskeratosis follicularis Darier. Заболевание наследуется аутосом но-доминантно, начинается в детском возрасте, характеризуется высыпанием мелких фолликулярных папул буровато-красноватого или серого цвета, покрытых плотно прилегающими корочка ми. Локализуются на коже лица (носогубные складки), шеи, гру ди, в межлопаточной области, в крупных складках кожи, а также на тыле кистей и стоп, где они очень сходны с плоскими бородав ками. Более редко могут встречаться буллезные и вегетирующие изменения.

Патогистология. Характерными гистологическими при знаками болезни Дарье являются своеобразная форма дискератоза с образованием круглых тел и зерен, надбазальный акантолиз, приводящий к появлению лакун, неравномерная пролиферация в лакунах сосочков дермы, окаймленных одним слоем базальных клеток, так называемые виллы. Наблюдаются также акантоз, па пилломатоз и гиперкератоз, а в собственно коже — хронический воспалительный инфильтрат (рис. 57). Круглые тела в централь ной части гомогенны, базофильны, окружены светлым ободком. В периферической части круглого тела (за ободком) находится базофильный дискератотический материал в виде оболочки. Не окрашенный ореол может быть замещен эозинофильным керато тическим материалом. Чем выше располагаются эти клетки в эпи дермисе, тем больше выражена в них кератинизация, исчезает ядро, однако базофильная зернистость часто сохраняется. Эти клетки можно видеть в щелях рогового слоя (рис. 58). Зерна в них менее заметны по сравнению с круглыми телами, они похожи на паракератотические клетки, но имеют более крупные удлиненные ядра, окруженные гомогенным дискератотическим материалом, окрашивающимся базофильно, реже — оксифильно. Лакуны — это маленькие щели, локализующиеся обычно внутриэпидермально, над базальным слоем. Они содержат акантолитические клетки, лишенные десмосом, с явлениями начинающейся кератинизации. Некоторые из них, сморщиваясь, становятся удлиненными и вы глядят аналогично зернам в роговом слое. Вследствие гиперкера тоза образуются роговые пробки. Выводные протоки потовых желез на всем протяжении как в дерме, так и в эпидермисе резко расширены, в отдельных местах нарушена целостность их стенок, в результате чего их просветы сообщаются с расщелинами между базальными и шиповатыми клетками эпидермиса.

В гипертрофических очагах отмечаются значительная пролифе рация эпидермиса по типу псевдоэпителиоматозной гиперплазии или появление узких отростков, состоящих из нескольких рядов базальных клеток, между которыми имеются узкие щели, или лакуны (рис. 59). Иногда в эпидермисе появляются пузырьки,

89

Figure 3.2. Page 89 from the textbook [2].

Example 2

The text on "Juvenile xanthogranuloma" on page 398 of the textbook Histopathology of the Skin by W.F. Lever and G. Schaumburg-Lever (Figure 3.3) reads as follows: "Histopathology. Early lesions may show large accumulations of histiocytes without any lipid infiltration intermingled with only a few lymphoid cells and eosinophils (Nödl; Gartmann and Tritsch). Usually, however, some degree of lipidization is present, even in very early lesions. One finds then in some of the histiocytes a pale, vacuolated cytoplasm staining positive with fat stains (Esterly et al). In mature lesions, a granulomatous infiltrate is usually present containing foam cells, foreign body giant cells, and Touton giant cells as well as histiocytes, lymphocytes, and eosinophils. The presence of giant cells, most of them Touton giant cells, showing a perfect "wreath" of nuclei is quite typical for juvenile xanthogranuloma (Gartmann and Tritsch; Webster et al). Older, regressing lesions show proliferation of fibroblasts and fibrosis replacing part of the infiltrate." [1]

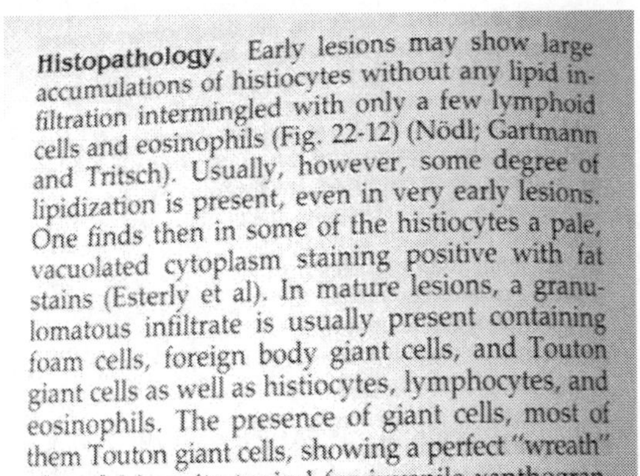

Histopathology. Early lesions may show large accumulations of histiocytes without any lipid infiltration intermingled with only a few lymphoid cells and eosinophils (Fig. 22-12) (Nödl; Gartmann and Tritsch). Usually, however, some degree of lipidization is present, even in very early lesions. One finds then in some of the histiocytes a pale, vacuolated cytoplasm staining positive with fat stains (Esterly et al). In mature lesions, a granulomatous infiltrate is usually present containing foam cells, foreign body giant cells, and Touton giant cells as well as histiocytes, lymphocytes, and eosinophils. The presence of giant cells, most of them Touton giant cells, showing a perfect "wreath" of nuclei is quite typical for juvenile xanthogranuloma (Fig. 22-13) (Gartmann and Tritsch; Webster et al). Older, regressing lesions show proliferation of fibroblasts and fibrosis replacing part of the infiltrate.

Figure 3.3. Juvenile xanthogranuloma. Reproduced from Lever's textbook Histopathology of the Skin, 1975 [1].

In the textbook by G.M. Tsvetkova and V.N. Mordovtsev (Figure 3.4), the text on page 107 can be translated in the following way: "Histopathology. Early lesions may show large accumulations of histiocytes or macrophages with lipid infiltration intermingled with only a few lymphoid cells and eosinophils. Lipidization can be seen even in very early lesions. One finds lipids among the histiocytes and macrophages, and also in the vacuolated cytoplasm of foam cells. In mature lesions, granulomatous foci are present, confluent with an infiltrate of foam cells, foreign body giant cells, and Touton giant cells as well as histiocytes, lymphocytes, and eosinophils. The presence of giant cells showing a wreath of nuclei is quite typical for juvenile xanthogranuloma. Older lesions show proliferation of fibroblasts and fibrosis" [2].

...цвета. С возрастом элементы спонтанно исчезают бесследно или оставляют после себя временную гиперпигментацию.

П а т о г и с т о л о г и я. В свежих очагах обнаруживают большое скопление гистиоцитов или макрофагов с инфильтрацией липидами и примесью небольшого числа лимфоидных клеток и эозинофильных гранулоцитов. Липидную инфильтрацию можно видеть и в очень ранних стадиях болезни. Липиды находятся среди гистиоцитов и макрофагов, а также в вакуолизированной цитоплазме пенистых клеток. В зрелых элементах имеются очаги гранулематозного строения, сливающиеся с инфильтратом из гистиоцитов, лимфоцитов, эозинофильных гранулоцитов, пенистых клеток и гигантских клеток типа Тутона. Среди них располагаются гигантские клетки, ядра которых размещены в виде венчика, что является типичным для ювенильной ксантогранулемы. В старых очагах отмечается пролиферация фибробластов и фиброз.

Ювенильную ксантогранулему дифференцируют от ранних стадий болезни Хенда—Шюллера—Крисчена, при которой выявляются массивные скопления мономорфных гистиоцитов, а также от ее гранулематозной стадии, дерматофибромы с липидизацией. При последней нет эозинофильных гранулоцитов и типичных для

Figure 3.4. Juvenile xanthogranuloma. Reproduced from [2].

Comment

The Russian text is somewhat shortened with deviations from the word-by-word translation. For example, the word "containing" was changed by the word with the meaning "confluent." However, the flow of the text and the sequence of sentences are identical to the original.

Example 3

The paragraph on "Xeroderma pigmentosum" on page 64 of the textbook by W.F. Lever and G. Schaumburg-Lever, shown in Figure 3.5, reads as follows: "Histopathology. In the early stage, the histopathological appearance is not specific, but the diagnosis is suggested by a combination of changes that normally are not seen in the skin of young persons. They are (1) hyperkeratosis, (2) thinning of the stratum malpighii with atrophy of some of the rete ridges and elongation of others, (3) a chronic inflammatory infiltrate in the upper dermis, and (4) irregular accumulations of melanin in the basal cell layer, either with or without an increase in the number of melanocytes present (Lynch et al, 1967).

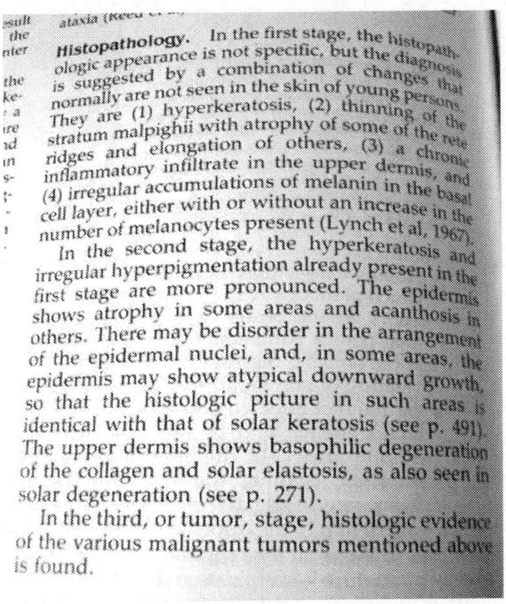

Histopathology. In the first stage, the histopathologic appearance is not specific, but the diagnosis is suggested by a combination of changes that normally are not seen in the skin of young persons. They are (1) hyperkeratosis, (2) thinning of the stratum malpighii with atrophy of some of the rete ridges and elongation of others, (3) a chronic inflammatory infiltrate in the upper dermis, and (4) irregular accumulations of melanin in the basal cell layer, either with or without an increase in the number of melanocytes present (Lynch et al, 1967).

In the second stage, the hyperkeratosis and irregular hyperpigmentation already present in the first stage are more pronounced. The epidermis shows atrophy in some areas and acanthosis in others. There may be disorder in the arrangement of the epidermal nuclei, and, in some areas, the epidermis may show atypical downward growth, so that the histologic picture in such areas is identical with that of solar keratosis (see p. 491). The upper dermis shows basophilic degeneration of the collagen and solar elastosis, as also seen in solar degeneration (see p. 271).

In the third, or tumor, stage, histologic evidence of the various malignant tumors mentioned above is found.

Figure 3.5. Xeroderma pigmentosum; reproduced from [1].

In the second stage, the hyperkeratosis and irregular hyperpigmentation already present in the first stage are more pronounced. The epidermis shows atrophy in some areas and acanthosis in others. There may be disorder in the arrangement of the epidermal nuclei, and, in some areas, the epidermis may show atypical downward growth, so that the histologic picture in such areas is identical with that of solar keratosis. The upper dermis shows basophilic degeneration of the collagen and solar elastosis, as also seen in solar degeneration" [1].

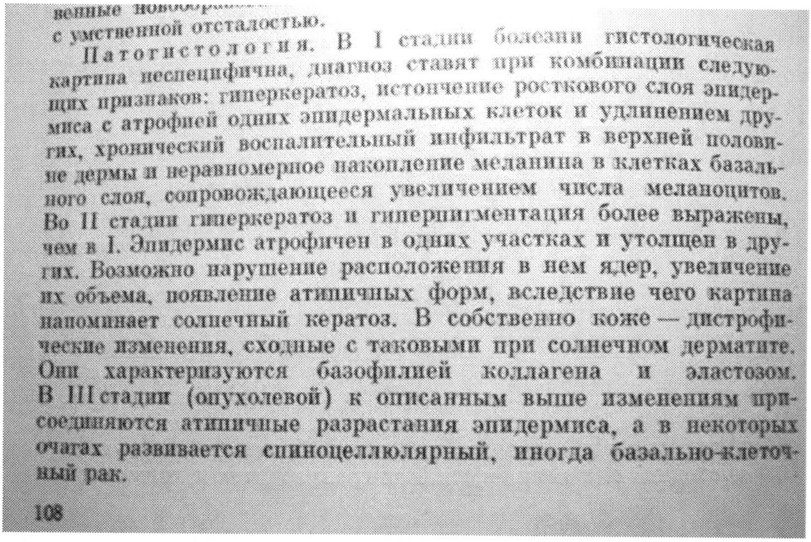
с умственной отсталостью.

Патогистология. В I стадии болезни гистологическая картина неспецифична, диагноз ставят при комбинации следующих признаков: гиперкератоз, истончение росткового слоя эпидермиса с атрофией одних эпидермальных клеток и удлинением других, хронический воспалительный инфильтрат в верхней половине дермы и неравномерное накопление меланина в клетках базального слоя, сопровождающееся увеличением числа меланоцитов. Во II стадии гиперкератоз и гиперпигментация более выражены, чем в I. Эпидермис атрофичен в одних участках и утолщен в других. Возможно нарушение расположения в нем ядер, увеличение их объема, появление атипичных форм, вследствие чего картина напоминает солнечный кератоз. В собственно коже — дистрофические изменения, сходные с таковыми при солнечном дерматите. Они характеризуются базофилией коллагена и эластозом. В III стадии (опухолевой) к описанным выше изменениям присоединяются атипичные разрастания эпидермиса, а в некоторых очагах развивается спиноцеллюлярный, иногда базально-клеточный рак.

108

Figure 3.6. Xeroderma pigmentosum. Reproduced from [2].

Figure 3.6 shows the text on the same subject on page 108 of the handbook G. Tsvetkova and V. Mordovtsev. It can be translated in the following way: "Histopathology. In the 1st stage of the disease, the histopathological appearance is not specific, but the diagnosis is suggested by a combination of the following signs: hyperkeratosis, thinning of the stratum malpighii with atrophy of some epidermal cells and elongation of others, a chronic inflammatory infiltrate in the upper half of the dermis, and irregular accumulations of melanin in the basal cell layer with an increase in the number of melanocytes present. In the 2nd stage, the hyperkeratosis and hyperpigmentation are more pronounced. The epidermis shows atrophy in some areas and thickening in others. There may be disorder in the arrangement of the epidermal nuclei, increase of their volume and appearance of atypical forms, so that the histologic picture resembles solar keratosis. The dermis shows dystrophic changes, similar to those in solar dermatitis. They are characterized by basophilia of the collagen and elastosis" [2].

Comment

The translation is shortened and there are some mistranslations, for example, the "atrophy of some of the rete ridges and elongation of others" was mistranslated as "atrophy of some epidermal cells and elongation of others." This mistranslation can be explained by the fact that the term "rete ridges" was absent in English-Russian dictionaries of that time and therefore was not known by all pathologists. Furthermore, the "upper dermis" was replaced by the "upper half of the dermis," which can be misleading because the upper dermis is a histological term, and its thickness does not necessarily mean a half of the dermal thickness. Finally, the term "solar elastosis" was replaced by "solar dermatitis" in the Russian edition, which is wrong because solar dermatitis develops with acute excessive sun exposure, while solar elastosis is a change in the connective tissue caused by chronic sun exposure being found, among others, in the skin of patients with xeroderma pigmentosum.

Example 4

In the Lever's textbook (Figure 3.7), the following is written on page 254 about "Sclerema neonatorum": "Histopathology. The subcutaneous tissue owes its thickening in sclerema neonatorum to an increase in the size of the fat cells and to the presence of wide, intersecting fibrous bands (Kellum et al). Many of the fat cells are filled with rosettes of fine, needlelike clefts. In frozen sections, these clefts are found to be occupied by crystals. The crystals fail to stain with fat stains but are doubly refractile in the polarizing microscope (Zeek and Madden). In most instances, there is no evidence of fat necrosis or inflammation (Kellum et al).

Histopathology. The subcutaneous tissue owes its thickening in sclerema neonatorum to an increase in the size of the fat cells and to the presence of wide, intersecting fibrous bands (Kellum et al). Many of the fat cells are filled with rosettes of fine, needlelike clefts. In frozen sections, these clefts are found to be occupied by crystals. The crystals fail to stain with fat stains but are doubly refractile in the polarizing microscope (Zeek and Madden). In most instances, there is no evidence of fat necrosis or inflammation (Kellum et al). In only some cases, one can see fat necrosis and an inflammatory reaction with giant cells (Zeek and Madden; Flory), but these changes are much less extensive and less pronounced than in subcutaneous fat necrosis of the newborn.

Systemic Lesions. In most cases of sclerema reported, the changes in the fatty tissue were found to be limited to the subcutaneous fat when an autopsy was performed (Kellum et al). In two cases of sclerema, however, autopsy revealed lesions in the visceral fat that were histologically identical with those observed in the subcutaneous fat. In one of these cases (Zeek and Madden), the lesions were widely distributed, whereas, in the other case (Flory), they were limited to the perirenal and retroperitoneal fat.

Histogenesis. The subcutaneous fat of the normal newborn, in comparison to adult subcutaneous fat, has greater amounts of saturated fatty acids, lower amounts of unsaturated fatty acids, a higher melting point, and a higher solidification point. The alterations in the subcutaneous fatty acids of infants with sclerema neonatorum represent an exaggeration of the normal newborn pattern. Thus, the increased ratio of saturated to unsaturated fatty acids in the subcutaneous triglycerides could be responsible for the physical changes of the subcutaneous fat in sclerema neonatorum (Kellum et al). The increased ratio of saturated to unsaturated fatty acids is probably due to defective enzyme mechanisms to unsaturate fatty acid chains (Kellum et al). As x-ray diffraction has shown, the doubly refractile crystals in the fat cells consist of triglycerides (Horsfield and Yardley).

Figure 3.7. Sclerema neonatorum. Reproduced from [1].

In only some cases, one can see fat necrosis and an inflammatory reaction with giant cells (Zeek and Madden; Flory), but these changes are much less extensive and less pronounced than in subcutaneous fat necrosis of the newborn.

Histogenesis. The subcutaneous fat of the normal newborn, in comparison to adult subcutaneous fat, has greater amount of saturated fatty acids, lower amounts of unsaturated fatty acids, a higher melting point, and a higher solidification point. The alterations in the subcutaneous fatty acids of infants with sclerema neonatorum represent an exaggeration of the normal newborn pattern. Thus, the increased ratio of saturated to unsaturated fatty acids in the subcutaneous triglycerides could be responsible for the physical changes of the subcutaneous fat in sclerema neonatorum (Kellum et al). The increased ratio of saturated to unsaturated fatty acids is probably due to defective enzyme mechanisms to unsaturate fatty acid chains (Kellum et al). As x-ray diffraction has shown, the doubly refractile crystals in the fat cells consist of triglycerides (Horsfield and Yardley)" [1].

The text from page 169 of the handbook [2] is shown in Figure 3.8. It can be translated as follows: "Histopathology. The subcutaneous tissue is thickened; fat cell groups in it are intersected by fibrous bands. Many of the fat cells are filled with rosettes or bundles of needlelike clefts. In frozen sections, these clefts are found to be occupied by crystals. The crystals stain positively with fat stains and are doubly refractile in the polarizing microscope. Sometimes one can see an inflammatory reaction with giant cells.

Histogenesis. The subcutaneous fat of the newborn, in comparison to adult subcutaneous fat, has greater amount of saturated fatty acids, lower amounts of unsaturated fatty acids, a higher melting point, and a higher solidification point. Thus, the increased ratio of saturated to unsaturated fatty acids in the subcutaneous triglycerides could be responsible for its physical changes (Kellium R. et al., 1968)... . As x-ray diffraction has shown, the doubly retractile crystals in the fat cells consist of triglycerides (Horsfield G., and Jardley H., 1965)" [2].

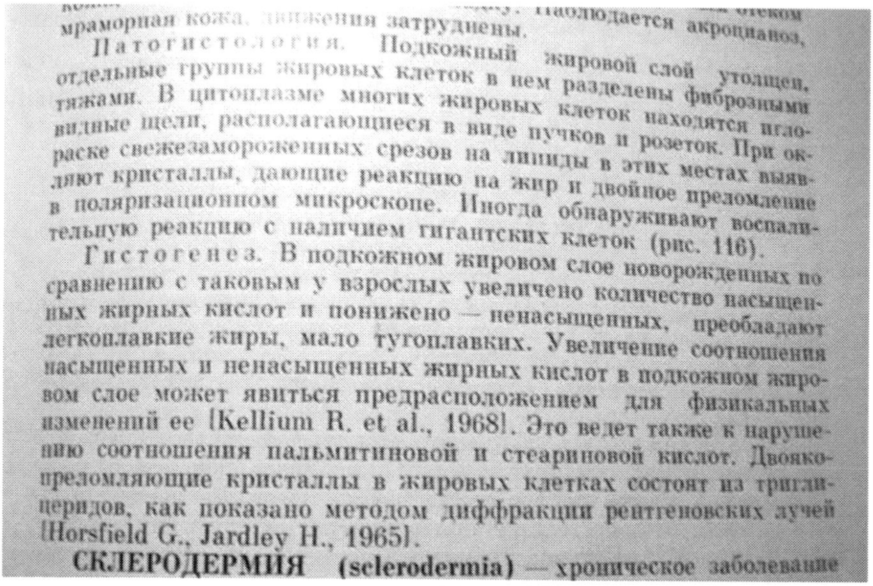

мраморная кожа, движения затруднены. Наблюдается акроцианоз,
Патогистология. Подкожный жировой слой утолщен,
отдельные группы жировых клеток в нем разделены фиброзными
тяжами. В цитоплазме многих жировых клеток находятся игло-
видные щели, располагающиеся в виде пучков и розеток. При ок-
раске свежезамороженных срезов на липиды в этих местах выяв-
ляют кристаллы, дающие реакцию на жир и двойное преломление
в поляризационном микроскопе. Иногда обнаруживают воспали-
тельную реакцию с наличием гигантских клеток (рис. 116).
Гистогенез. В подкожном жировом слое новорожденных по
сравнению с таковым у взрослых увеличено количество насыщен-
ных жирных кислот и понижено — ненасыщенных, преобладают
легкоплавкие жиры, мало тугоплавких. Увеличение соотношения
насыщенных и ненасыщенных жирных кислот в подкожном жиро-
вом слое может явиться предрасположением для физикальных
изменений ее [Kellium R. et al., 1968]. Это ведет также к наруше-
нию соотношения пальмитиновой и стеариновой кислот. Двояко-
преломляющие кристаллы в жировых клетках состоят из тригли-
церидов, как показано методом дифракции рентгеновских лучей
[Horsfield G., Jardley H., 1965].
СКЛЕРОДЕРМИЯ (sclerodermia) — хроническое заболевание

Figure 3.8. Sclerema neonatorum; reproduced from [2].

Comment

The text in Russian language is shorter compared to the original text in the Lever's textbook. The translation also has a few additions and inaccuracies. As an example, in the original it says "the crystals fail to stain with fat stains" while the Russian edition notes that they "stain with fat stains." Most probably, it is negligence of translation. Considering that the crystals are breakdown products of fat such as sodium stearate and palmitic acid, they must be negative with usual fat stains, where the dye is dissolved by triglycerides. For example, Sudan Black, one of the most popular of all Sudan dyes, fails to stain crystalline lipids and free fatty acids [3, 4]. Of note is also that the Russian text includes only two of the four references given in Lever's textbook whereas one author's name is misspelled (Figure 3.8).

Example 5

Histopathology. *Solitary glomus tumors* are surrounded by a fibrous capsule. They contain numerous small vascular lumina that are lined by a single layer of flattened, often elongated endothelial cells. Peripheral to the endothelial cells are a few to many layers of glomus cells (Fig. 30-7). The glomus cells have a faintly eosinophilic cytoplasm and large, pale, round to oval nuclei of a rather uniform appearance. The glomus cells thus resemble epithelioid cells. In many areas, the glomus cells are seen to extend irregularly from the vascular walls into the connective tissue stroma of the tumor. This stroma appears edematous and contains scattered fibroblasts and fairly numerous mast cells (Murad et al). Staining with the Bodian stain shows a considerable number of nerve fibers in the perivascular stroma of solitary tumors (Shugart et al).

Multiple glomus tumors possess no capsule and show much larger vascular spaces than the solitary glomus tumor. Because of their conspicuous vascular component, multiple glomus tumors are referred to also as *glomangiomas* (Laymon and Peterson). The large vascular spaces usually have an irregular shape. Just as in the solitary glomus tumor, the vascular spaces are lined by a single layer of flat endothelial cells, but the number of glomus cells located peripheral to the endothelial cells is much smaller than in the solitary glomus tumor (Fig. 30-8). Usually, the glomus cells form only a narrow rim of one to three layers. They may even be absent around part of the vessel walls, and some of the vascular spaces may show no glomus cells (Laymon and Peterson). Rarely, a patient may show glomus cells in only some of his tumors and none in others (Schnyder). With the Bodian stain, only few nerve fibers are seen in the connective tissue surrounding the vascular formations of multiple glomus tumors (Gordon and Hyman; Chandon et al).

Figure 3.9. Glomus tumor; reproduced from [1].

Walter F. Lever and Gundula Schaumburg-Lever comment on page 633 of their textbook on "Glomus tumor" (Figure 3.9): "Histopathology. Solitary glomus tumors are surrounded by a fibrous capsule. They contain numerous small vascular lumina that are lined by a single layer of flattened, often elongated endothelial cells. Peripheral to the endothelial cells are a few to many layers of glomus cells. The glomus cells have a faintly eosinophilic cytoplasm and large, pale round to oval nuclei of a rather uniform appearance. The glomus cells thus resemble epithelioid cells. In many areas, the glomus cells are seen to extend irregularly from the vascular walls... .

> "Multiple glomus tumors possess no capsule and show much larger vascular spaces than the solitary glomus tumor. Because of their conspicuous vascular component, multiple glomus tumors are referred to as glomangiomas (Laymon and Peterson). The large vascular spaces usually have an irregular shape. Just as in the solitary glomus tumor, the vascular spaces are lined by a single layer of flat endothelial cells, but the number of glomus cells located peripheral to the endothelial cells is much smaller than in the solitary glomus tumor. Usually, the glomus cells form only a narrow rim of one or three layers. They may even be absent..." [1].

The text on the same tumor on page 219 of the handbook [4] by Galina Tsvetkova and Vladimir Mordovtsev (Figure 3.10) can be translated as follows: "Histopathology. A solitary nodule of a glomus-angioma contains numerous small vascular lumina that are lined by a single layer of flattened endothelial cells. Peripheral to the endothelial cells are a few to many layers of glomus cells having a faintly eosinophilic cytoplasm and large, dark round to oval nuclei resembling epithelial elements. In many areas, the glomus cells are seen to extend irregularly from the vascular walls, their polymorphism and dystrophic changes can be seen.

Multiple glomus-angiomas possess no capsule and show much larger vascular spaces. The large vascular spaces usually have an irregular shape. Just as in the solitary nodule, the vascular spaces are lined by a single layer of flat endothelial cells, but the number of glomus cells located peripheral to the endothelial cells is much smaller, they form only a narrow rim of 2 layers. They may not visible at all" [2].

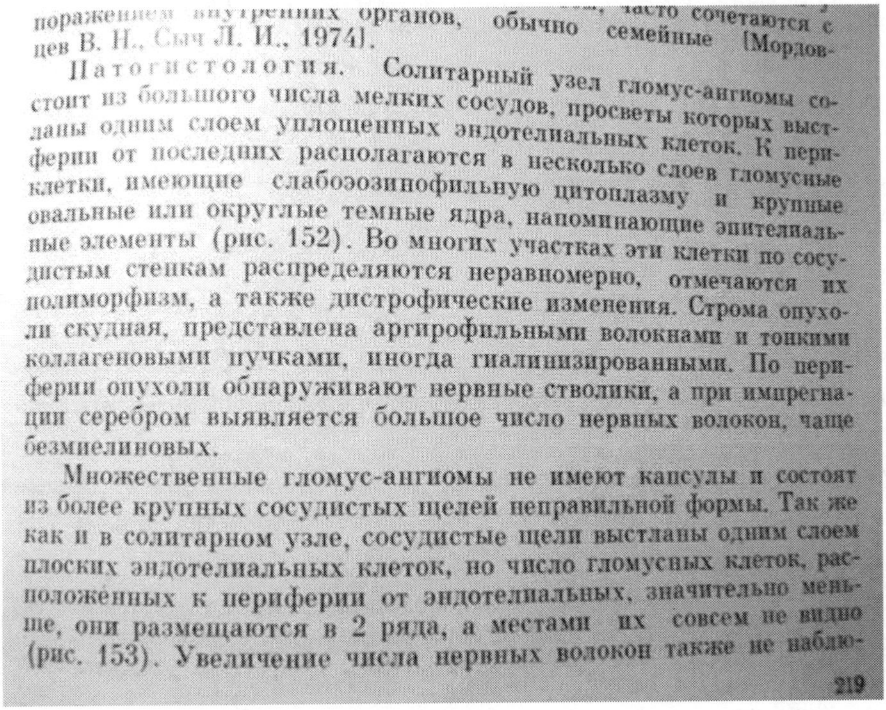

поражением внутренних органов, обычно семейные ..., часто сочетаются с ... [Мордовцев В. Н., Сыч Л. И., 1974].

Патогистология. Солитарный узел гломус-ангиомы состоит из большого числа мелких сосудов, просветы которых выстланы одним слоем уплощенных эндотелиальных клеток. К периферии от последних располагаются в несколько слоев гломусные клетки, имеющие слабоэозинофильную цитоплазму и крупные овальные или округлые темные ядра, напоминающие эпителиальные элементы (рис. 152). Во многих участках эти клетки по сосудистым стенкам распределяются неравномерно, отмечаются их полиморфизм, а также дистрофические изменения. Строма опухоли скудная, представлена аргирофильными волокнами и тонкими коллагеновыми пучками, иногда гиалинизированными. По периферии опухоли обнаруживают нервные стволики, а при импрегнации серебром выявляется большое число нервных волокон, чаще безмиелиновых.

Множественные гломус-ангиомы не имеют капсулы и состоят из более крупных сосудистых щелей неправильной формы. Так же как и в солитарном узле, сосудистые щели выстланы одним слоем плоских эндотелиальных клеток, но число гломусных клеток, расположённых к периферии от эндотелиальных, значительно меньше, они размещаются в 2 ряда, а местами их совсем не видно (рис. 153). Увеличение числа нервных волокон также не наблю-

219

Figure 3.10. Glomus tumor; reproduced from [2].

Comment

The Russian text, once again, is shorter compared with the Lever's text, and it is inaccurate in places e.g., "epithelioid" is translated as "epithelial." An addition about cytomorphology of glomus cells is made by the Russian authors: "Their polymorphism and dystrophic changes can be seen" [2]. This, however, is misleading because cells in glomus tumors are usually rather uniform; their nuclei show a bland chromatin pattern with inconspicuous to well-defined nucleoli. Rarely, when glomus tumors exhibit large pleomorphic nuclei without other high-grade histologic features, such as increased cellularity and multiple mitoses, they are referred to as symplastic glomus tumors. Otherwise, in combination with the increased mitotic rate or the presence of atypical mitotic figures, a moderate-to-high nuclear grade should be regarded as an indication to a possibly malignant character or an uncertain malignant potential of a glomus tumor [5-7]. Therefore, the addition made by Tsvetkova and Mordovtsev to the original description can be misleading for a practitioner.

CONCLUSION

It should not be left without comment, when the celebrated editions such as Lever's Histopathology of the Skin, Robbins' Pathologic Basis of Disease, Enzinger's Soft Tissue Tumors, or the Handbuch der Speziellen Pathologischen Anatomie und Histologie by Henke and Lubarsch (discussed in Chapter 6), are rewritten without proper references, mistranslated, and distorted by additions. We can hardly imagine what immense work and immaculate integrity stands behind these great and truthful books. These works and their authors deserve to be treated with respect by exact quotations and references. Today's and tomorrow's plagiarists should be aware that they may be identified and exposed. Otherwise the misconduct would spread over the globe and persist endlessly.

REFERENCES

[1] Lever WF, Schaumburg-Lever G. *Lever's Histopathology of the Skin.* Philadelphia: Lippincott, 1975.

[2] Tsvetkova GM, Mordovtsev VN. *Patomorfologicheskaya diagnostika zabolevanii kozhi [Pathomorphologic Diagnosis of Skin Diseases]*. Moscow: Meditsina, 1986.

[3] Proks C, Valvoda V. Fatty crystals in sclerema neonatorum. *J Clin Pathol* 1966;19(2):193-5.

[4] Bayliss High OB. The histochemical versatility of Sudan Black B. *Acta Histochem Suppl* 1981;24:247-55.

[5] Gombos Z, Zhang PJ. Glomus tumor. *Arch Pathol Lab Med* 2008;132(9):1448-52.

[6] Khoury T, Balos L, McGrath B, Wong MK, Cheney RT, Tan D. Malignant glomus tumor: a case report and review of literature, focusing on its clinicopathologic features and immunohistochemical profile. *Am J Dermatopathol* 2005;27(5):428-31.

[7] Kayal JD, Hampton RW, Sheehan DJ, Washington CV. Malignant glomus tumor: a case report and review of the literature. *Dermatol Surg* 2001;27(9):837-40.

Chapter 4

HOW TO WRITE A TEXTBOOK FROM THE INTERNET

In a textbook by Trufanov and Fokin titled Magnetic Resonance Tomography, Handbook for Physicians (in Russian) [1], entire paragraphs were copied from other sources without references (Figure 4.1).

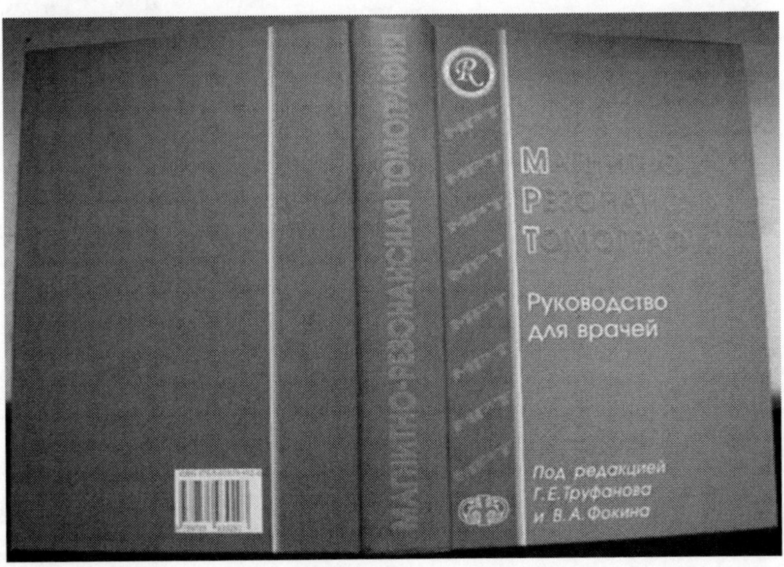

Figure 4.1. Cover of the textbook [1].

Apparently, the text was translated from English not by doctors but by professional translators insufficiently acquainted with the medical terminology. It is known that some translating firms in Moscow were overloaded by medical texts. In the text of this handbook many English medical terms are transliterated into Cyrillic alphabet instead of using Russian equivalents known by physicians. Mistranslations can be encountered as well.

We have found three sources of the borrowing: an open access website [2] and two books partly available online as free previews [3, 4]. Neither of these sources was mentioned in the reference list of the handbook [1].

The chapter of the manual [1] "History of emergence and development of magnetic resonance imaging" (pp. 11-26) is partly represented by a translation with large fragments taken verbatim from the website EMRF online [2]. Figure 4.2a,b are screenshots from this website; Figure 4.2c,d are photographs of corresponding pages of the handbook [1].

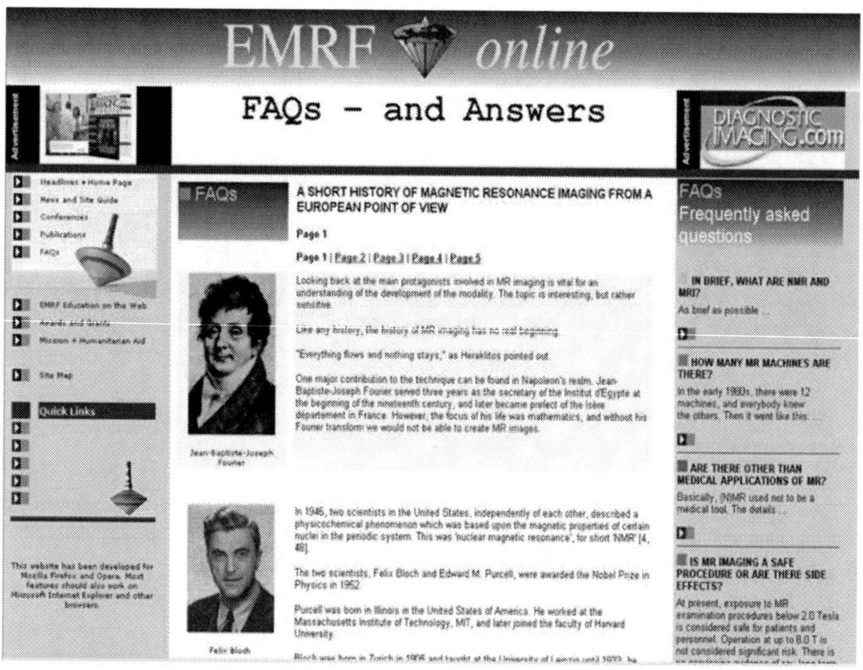

a)

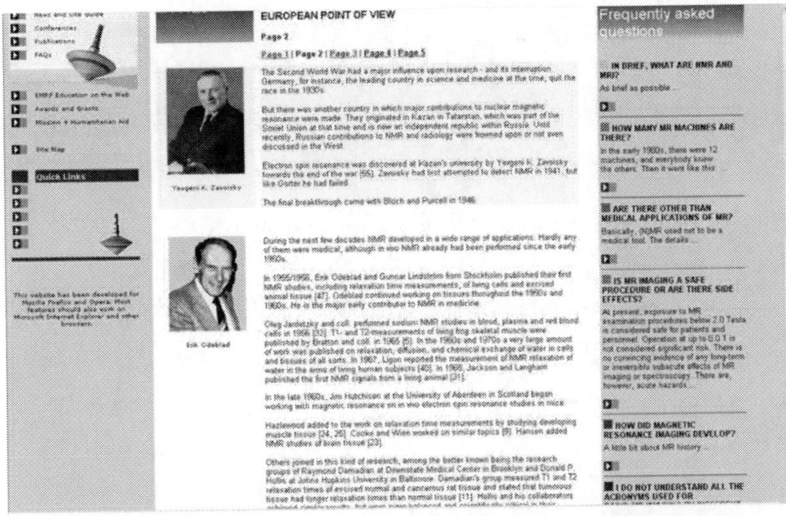

b)

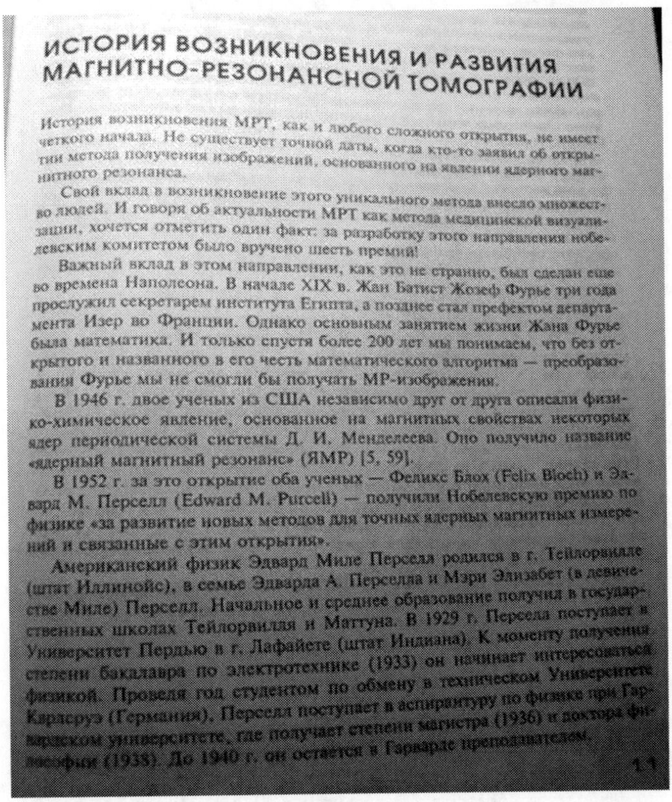

ИСТОРИЯ ВОЗНИКНОВЕНИЯ И РАЗВИТИЯ МАГНИТНО-РЕЗОНАНСНОЙ ТОМОГРАФИИ

История возникновения МРТ, как и любого сложного открытия, не имеет четкого начала. Не существует точной даты, когда кто-то заявил об открытии метода получения изображений, основанного на явлении ядерного магнитного резонанса.

Свой вклад в возникновение этого уникального метода внесло множество людей. И говоря об актуальности МРТ как метода медицинской визуализации, хочется отметить один факт: за разработку этого направления нобелевским комитетом было вручено шесть премий!

Важный вклад в этом направлении, как это не странно, был сделан еще во времена Наполеона. В начале XIX в. Жан Батист Жозеф Фурье три года прослужил секретарем института Египта, а позднее стал префектом департамента Изер во Франции. Однако основным занятием жизни Жана Фурье была математика. И только спустя более 200 лет мы понимаем, что без открытого и названного в его честь математического алгоритма — преобразования Фурье мы не смогли бы получать МР-изображения.

В 1946 г. двое ученых из США независимо друг от друга описали физико-химическое явление, основанное на магнитных свойствах некоторых ядер периодической системы Д. И. Менделеева. Оно получило название «ядерный магнитный резонанс» (ЯМР) [5, 59].

В 1952 г. за это открытие оба ученых — Феликс Блох (Felix Bloch) и Эдвард М. Перселл (Edward M. Purcell) — получили Нобелевскую премию по физике «за развитие новых методов для точных ядерных магнитных измерений и связанные с этим открытия».

Американский физик Эдвард Миле Перселл родился в г. Тейлорвилле (штат Иллинойс), в семье Эдварда А. Перселла и Мэри Элизабет (в девичестве Миле) Перселл. Начальное и среднее образование получил в государственных школах Тейлорвилля и Маттуна. В 1929 г. Перселл поступает в Университет Пердью в г. Лафайете (штат Индиана). К моменту получения степени бакалавра по электротехнике (1933) он начинает интересоваться физикой. Проведя год студентом по обмену в техническом Университете Карлсруэ (Германия), Перселл поступает в аспирантуру по физике при Гарвардском университете, где получает степени магистра (1936) и доктора философии (1938). До 1940 г. он остается в Гарварде преподавателем.

11

c)

Figure 4.2. (Continued).

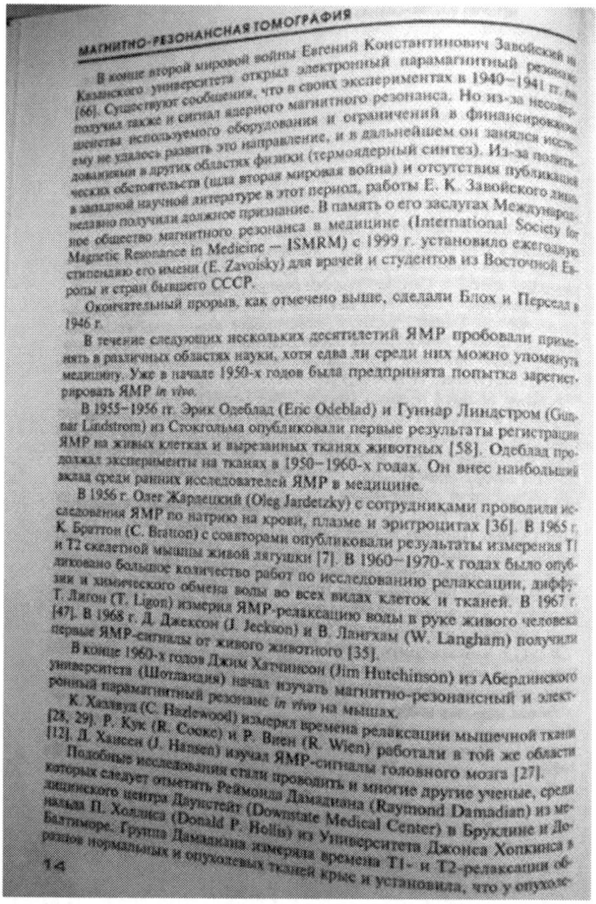

МАГНИТНО-РЕЗОНАНСНАЯ ТОМОГРАФИЯ

В конце второй мировой войны Евгений Константинович Завойский из
Казанского университета открыл электронный парамагнитный резонанс
[66]. Существуют сообщения, что в своих экспериментах в 1940–1941 гг. он
получил также и сигнал ядерного магнитного резонанса. Но из-за несовер-
шенства используемого оборудования и ограничений в финансировании
ему не удалось развить это направление, и в дальнейшем он занялся иссле-
дованиями в других областях физики (термоядерный синтез). Из-за полити-
ческих обстоятельств (шла вторая мировая война) и отсутствия публикаций
в западной научной литературе в этот период, работы Е. К. Завойского лишь
недавно получили должное признание. В память о его заслугах Международ-
ное общество магнитного резонанса в медицине (International Society for
Magnetic Resonance in Medicine — ISMRM) с 1999 г. установило ежегодную
стипендию его имени (E. Zavoisky) для врачей и студентов из Восточной Ев-
ропы и стран бывшего СССР.

Окончательный прорыв, как отмечено выше, сделали Блох и Перселл в
1946 г.

В течение следующих нескольких десятилетий ЯМР пробовали приме-
нять в различных областях науки, хотя едва ли среди них можно упомянуть
медицину. Уже в начале 1950-х годов была предпринята попытка зарегист-
рировать ЯМР *in vivo*.

В 1955–1956 гг. Эрик Одеблад (Eric Odeblad) и Гуннар Линдстром (Gun-
nar Lindstrom) из Стокгольма опубликовали первые результаты регистрации
ЯМР на живых клетках и вырезанных тканях животных [58]. Одеблад про-
должал эксперименты на тканях в 1950–1960-х годах. Он внес наибольший
вклад среди ранних исследователей ЯМР в медицине.

В 1956 г. Олег Жарецкий (Oleg Jardetzky) с сотрудниками проводили ис-
следования ЯМР по натрию на крови, плазме и эритроцитах [36]. В 1965 г.
К. Браттон (C. Bratton) с соавторами опубликовали результаты измерения T1
и T2 скелетной мышцы живой лягушки [7]. В 1960–1970-х годах было опуб-
ликовано большое количество работ по исследованию релаксации, диффу-
зии и химического обмена воды во всех видах клеток и тканей. В 1967 г.
Г. Лигон (T. Ligon) измерил ЯМР-релаксацию воды в руке живого человека
[47]. В 1968 г. Д. Джексон (J. Jeckson) и В. Лангхам (W. Langham) получили
первые ЯМР-сигналы от живого животного [35].

В конце 1960-х годов Джим Хатчинсон (Jim Hutchinson) из Абердинского
университета (Шотландия) начал изучать магнитно-резонансный и элект-
ронный парамагнитный резонанс *in vivo* на мышах.

К. Хазлвуд (C. Hazlewood) измерил времена релаксации мышечной ткани
[28, 29]. Р. Кук (R. Cooke) и Р. Виен (R. Wien) работали в той же области
[12]. Д. Хансен (J. Hansen) изучал ЯМР-сигналы головного мозга [27].

Подобные исследования стали проводить и многие другие ученые, среди
которых следует отметить Реймонда Дамадиана (Raymond Damadian) из ме-
дицинского центра Даунстейт (Downstate Medical Center) в Бруклине и До-
нальда П. Холлиса (Donald P. Hollis) из Университета Джонса Хопкинса в
Балтиморе. Группа Дамадиана измеряла времена T1- и T2-релаксации об-
разцов нормальных и опухолевых тканей крыс и установила, что у опухоле-

14

d)

Figure 4.2a,b. a - Screenshots from the [2]; c,d - Corresponding pages from the textbook [1].

From a textbook titled Clinical Cardiac MRI by Bogaert, Dymarkovski, and Taylor, the borrowed text was found in the chapter “MRI diagnostics of ischemic and non-ischemic diseases of myocardium” (pp. 370-413) [3]. Figure 4.3a,b are copies of the section “Cardiac Hypertrophy” from both editions. The whole section was borrowed verbatim. Other sections were available online as a free preview (“Restrictive cardiomyopathy,” “Amyloidosis,” etc.) and were borrowed verbatim from this source. Numerical data from these sections are transferred without change to the Russian handbook.

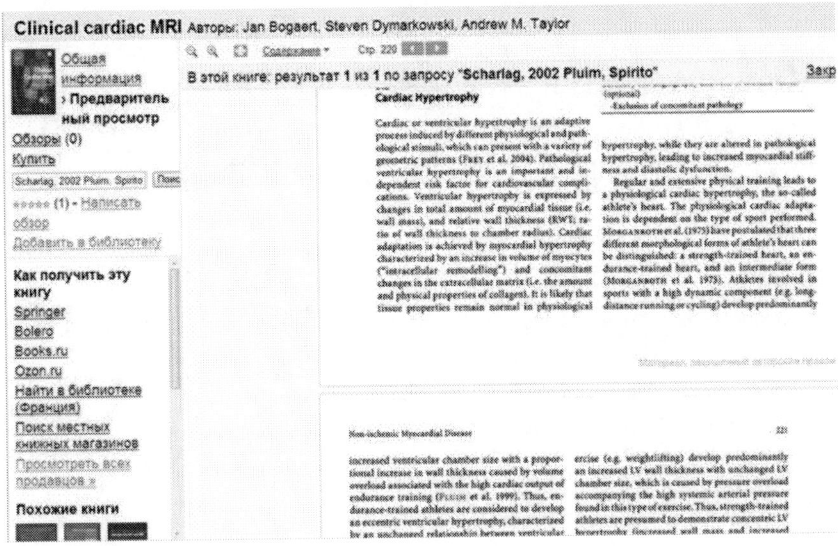

a)

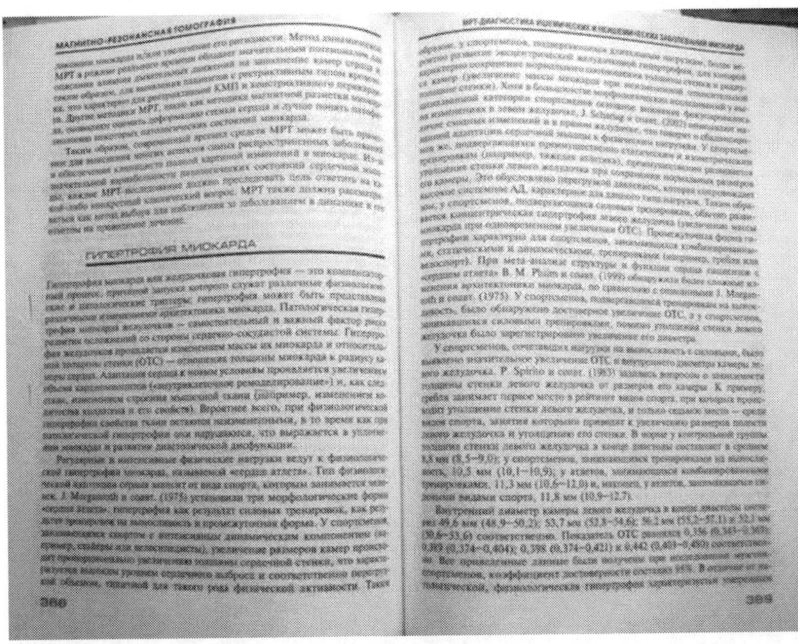

b)

Figure 4.3a,b. a - Page 220 from the book [3], section Cardiac Hypertrophy; b - pages 388-389 from the book [1], section Cardiac Hypertrophy.

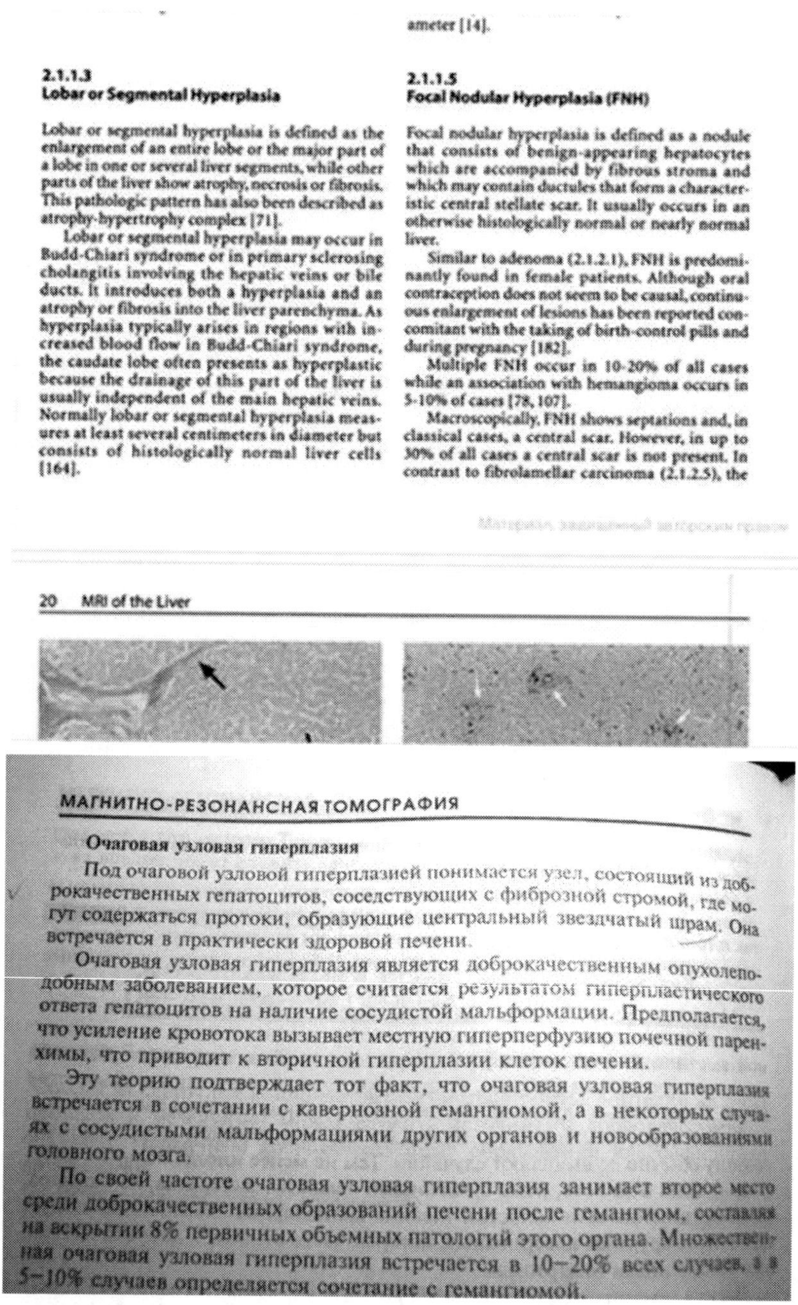

ameter [14].

2.1.1.3
Lobar or Segmental Hyperplasia

Lobar or segmental hyperplasia is defined as the enlargement of an entire lobe or the major part of a lobe in one or several liver segments, while other parts of the liver show atrophy, necrosis or fibrosis. This pathologic pattern has also been described as atrophy-hypertrophy complex [71].

Lobar or segmental hyperplasia may occur in Budd-Chiari syndrome or in primary sclerosing cholangitis involving the hepatic veins or bile ducts. It introduces both a hyperplasia and an atrophy or fibrosis into the liver parenchyma. As hyperplasia typically arises in regions with increased blood flow in Budd-Chiari syndrome, the caudate lobe often presents as hyperplastic because the drainage of this part of the liver is usually independent of the main hepatic veins. Normally lobar or segmental hyperplasia measures at least several centimeters in diameter but consists of histologically normal liver cells [164].

2.1.1.5
Focal Nodular Hyperplasia (FNH)

Focal nodular hyperplasia is defined as a nodule that consists of benign-appearing hepatocytes which are accompanied by fibrous stroma and which may contain ductules that form a characteristic central stellate scar. It usually occurs in an otherwise histologically normal or nearly normal liver.

Similar to adenoma (2.1.2.1), FNH is predominantly found in female patients. Although oral contraception does not seem to be causal, continuous enlargement of lesions has been reported concomitant with the taking of birth-control pills and during pregnancy [182].

Multiple FNH occur in 10-20% of all cases while an association with hemangioma occurs in 5-10% of cases [78, 107].

Macroscopically, FNH shows septations and, in classical cases, a central scar. However, in up to 30% of all cases a central scar is not present. In contrast to fibrolamellar carcinoma (2.1.2.5), the

20 MRI of the Liver

a)

МАГНИТНО-РЕЗОНАНСНАЯ ТОМОГРАФИЯ

Очаговая узловая гиперплазия

Под очаговой узловой гиперплазией понимается узел, состоящий из доброкачественных гепатоцитов, соседствующих с фиброзной стромой, где могут содержаться протоки, образующие центральный звездчатый шрам. Она встречается в практически здоровой печени.

Очаговая узловая гиперплазия является доброкачественным опухолеподобным заболеванием, которое считается результатом гиперпластического ответа гепатоцитов на наличие сосудистой мальформации. Предполагается, что усиление кровотока вызывает местную гиперперфузию почечной паренхимы, что приводит к вторичной гиперплазии клеток печени.

Эту теорию подтверждает тот факт, что очаговая узловая гиперплазия встречается в сочетании с кавернозной гемангиомой, а в некоторых случаях с сосудистыми мальформациями других органов и новообразованиями головного мозга.

По своей частоте очаговая узловая гиперплазия занимает второе место среди доброкачественных образований печени после гемангиом, составляя на вскрытии 8% первичных объемных патологий этого органа. Множественная очаговая узловая гиперплазия встречается в 10–20% всех случаев, а в 5–10% случаев определяется сочетание с гемангиомой.

b)

Figure 4.4a,b. a - Page 19 from the book [4], section Focal Nodular Hyperplasia; b - Page 438 from the book [1], section Focal Nodular Hyperplasia.

The chapter "MRI diagnostics of liver, gallbladder and biliary tract diseases" (pp. 429-485) has its own source, namely, a textbook [4]. Some paragraphs are copied verbatim as well, but the Russian text differs somewhat more from the original. At the same time, mistranslations have been found here, leading to the distortion of the meaning. Some examples are given below:

Figure 4.4a,b show the first paragraph, translated verbatim. The word "scar" is translated into Russian as "shram," which is not a medical term but a colloquial word with the meaning "posttraumatic scar of the skin". This demonstrates an unprofessional quality of the translation.

2.1.2.4
Hepatocellular Carcinoma (HCC)

In Europe and North America the incidence of HCC is generally below 3/100,000 inhabitants, while in parts of Asia and Africa it is about thirty times higher. The endemic occurrence of chronic hepatitis B and exposure to Aflatoxin B1 seem to be primary reasons for this [8]. In Europe and Japan the leading cause of HCC is chronic hepatitis C with consecutive cirrhosis [53].

Patients with chronic hepatitis or hemochromatosis have the highest risk of developing HCC. On the other hand, alcohol-induced cirrhosis, autoimmune hepatitis and α-1-antitrypsin-deficiency do not seem to increase the risk significantly. Similarly, primary biliary cirrhosis and Wilson's disease do not predispose subjects to an increased incidence of HCC [135].

Generally, the prognosis for patients with HCC is poor, and is largely dependent upon the extent of surgical intervention, the size of tumor growth, the functionality of the remaining liver parenchyma and the possibility of infiltration of the portal vein [199] (Fig. 12).

Whereas the ultimate procedure for the potential cure of patients with HCC remains liver transplantation [153], possibilities for palliative treatment include intraarterial injection of ^{131}Iod-Lipiodol or alcohol [55].

The macropathological division of HCC, which dates from the beginning of the 20th century, correlates relatively well with imaging findings. Three main types can be distinguished:

- the multinodular type with multiple, sharply-demarcated tumor nodules,
- the massive type with one single tumor node and smaller satellite nodules,
- the diffuse type with tumor areas interspersed throughout the liver.

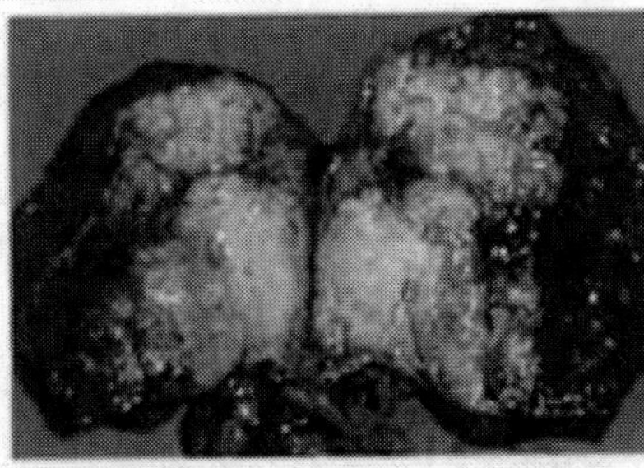

Fig. 12. Cut surface of a hepatocellular carcinoma without a capsule, infiltrating the liver parenchyma

small but significant (about 7%) proportion of cases [100].

A proposal as to how the multi-step development of HCC can be interpreted is presented in Table 1. However, it is important to realize that reliable differentiation between pre-cancerous developments, such as high-grade dysplastic nodules, and well-differentiated HCC is not always possible [58, 142].

Microscopically, HCC has several patterns. HCC is composed of malignant hepatocytes that differentiate into normal liver structures and mimic normal hepatocyte growth, but do not form normal hepatic acini (Fig. 13). Cells in well-differentiated HCC are difficult to distinguish from normal hepatocytes or hepatocellular adenoma cells. Malignant hepatocytes may even produce bile (Fig. 14). In other cases, there are microscopic variations, with HCC containing fat (Fig. 15), tumoral secretions (large amounts of watery material), fibrosis, necrosis and amorphous calcifications (Figs. 16, 17). This variable microscopic presenta- a)

Figure 4.5. (Continued).

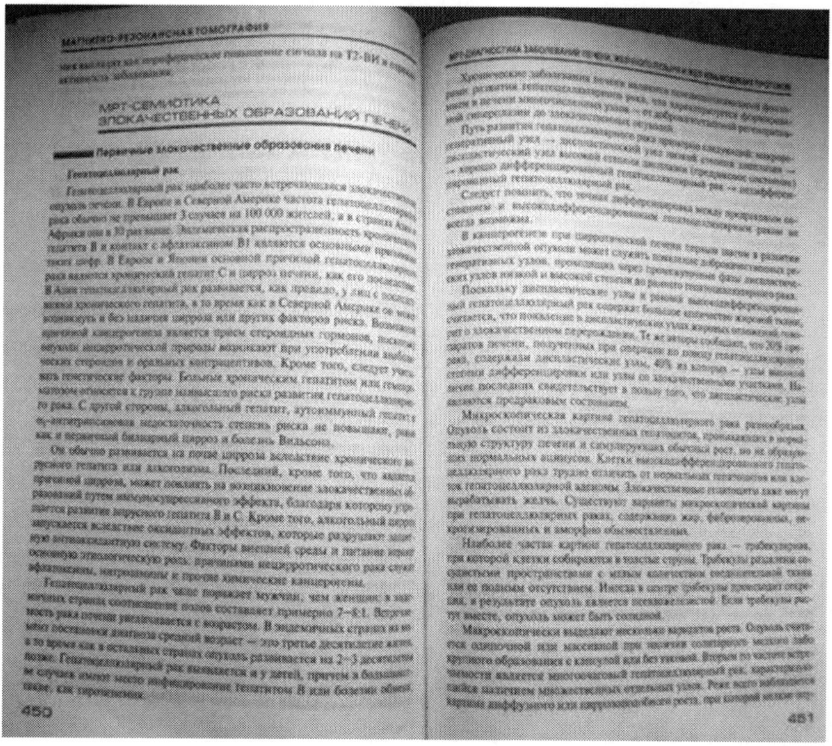
МАГНИТНО-РЕЗОНАНСНАЯ ТОМОГРАФИЯ

МРТ-СЕМИОТИКА ЗЛОКАЧЕСТВЕННЫХ ОБРАЗОВАНИЙ ПЕЧЕНИ

Первичные злокачественные образования печени

Гепатоцеллюлярный рак

450

451

b)

Figure 4.5a,b. a - Page 23 from the book [4], section Hepatocellular Carcinoma; b - Pages 450-451 from the book [1], section Hepatocellular Carcinoma.

In Figures 4-5a,b, the first and the last paragraphs about hepatocellular carcinoma (HCC) are copied verbatim. The translated fragment reads: “Microscopically, HCC has several patterns. HCC is composed of malignant hepatocytes that differentiate into normal liver structures and mimic normal hepatocyte growth, but do not form normal hepatic acini. Cells in well-differentiated HCC are difficult to distinguish from normal hepatocytes or of normal hepatocellular adenoma cells. Malignant hepatocytes can even produce bile. In other cases, there are microscopic variations, with HCC containing fat, tumoral secretions (large amounts of watery material), fibrosis, necrosis and amorphous calcifications” [1]. It contains a mistranslation with an alteration of the meaning: the phrase “hepatocytes that differentiate into normal liver structures” [4] is mistranslated into “hepatocytes that penetrate into normal liver structure” [1].

Figure 4.6a,b shows a section on “Fibrolammelar carcinoma” (FLC), which is copied almost entirely verbatim. A mistranslation significant for a histopathologist can be found in the phrase “FLC lesions have a distinctive microscopic pattern and are composed of eosinophilic, malignant hepatocytes containing prominent nuclei.” The professional term “prominent nuclei” is mistranslated by a word with the meaning “clear” or “clearly visible” nuclei.

It should be pointed out in conclusion that the MRI handbook [1], officially recommended for postgraduate training of physicians, is relatively expensive in comparison with similar Russian editions.

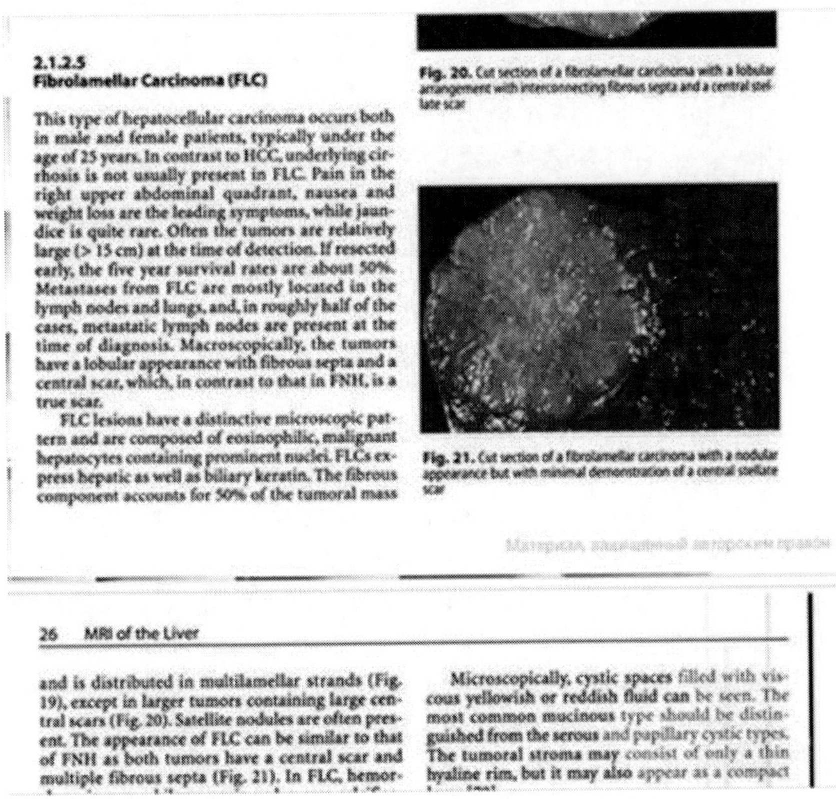

2.1.2.5
Fibrolamellar Carcinoma (FLC)

This type of hepatocellular carcinoma occurs both in male and female patients, typically under the age of 25 years. In contrast to HCC, underlying cirrhosis is not usually present in FLC. Pain in the right upper abdominal quadrant, nausea and weight loss are the leading symptoms, while jaundice is quite rare. Often the tumors are relatively large (> 15 cm) at the time of detection. If resected early, the five year survival rates are about 50%. Metastases from FLC are mostly located in the lymph nodes and lungs, and, in roughly half of the cases, metastatic lymph nodes are present at the time of diagnosis. Macroscopically, the tumors have a lobular appearance with fibeous septa and a central scar, which, in contrast to that in FNH, is a true scar.

FLC lesions have a distinctive microscopic pattern and are composed of eosinophilic, malignant hepatocytes containing prominent nuclei. FLCs express hepatic as well as biliary keratin. The fibrous component accounts for 50% of the tumoral mass

Fig. 20. Cut section of a fibrolamellar carcinoma with a lobular arrangement with interconnecting fibrous septa and a central stellate scar

Fig. 21. Cut section of a fibrolamellar carcinoma with a nodular appearance but with minimal demonstration of a central stellate scar

26 MRI of the Liver

and is distributed in multilamellar strands (Fig. 19), except in larger tumors containing large central scars (Fig. 20). Satellite nodules are often present. The appearance of FLC can be similar to that of FNH as both tumors have a central scar and multiple fibrous septa (Fig. 21). In FLC, hemor-

Microscopically, cystic spaces filled with viscous yellowish or reddish fluid can be seen. The most common mucinous type should be distinguished from the serous and papillary cystic types. The tumoral stroma may consist of only a thin hyaline rim, but it may also appear as a compact

a)

Figure 4.6. (Continued).

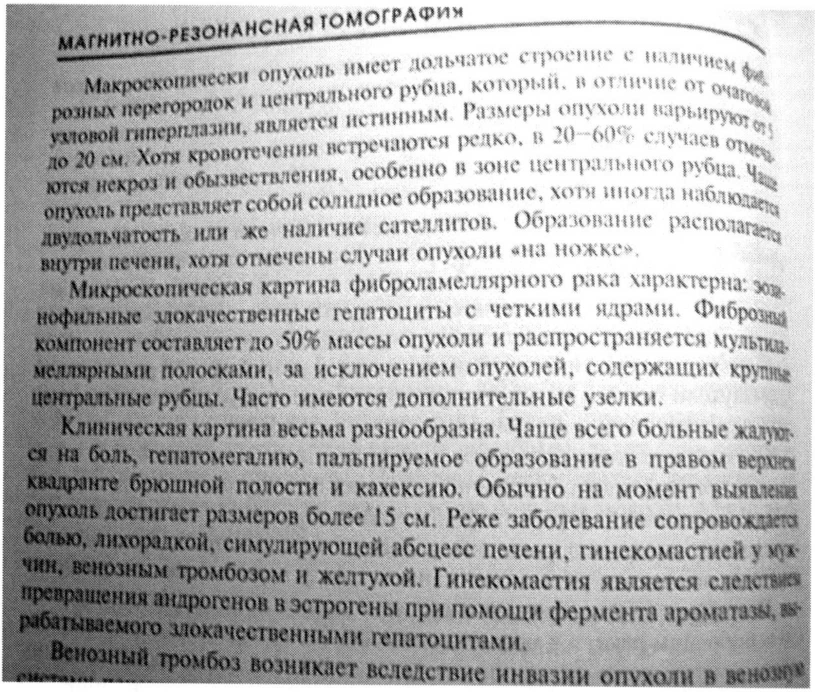

МАГНИТНО-РЕЗОНАНСНАЯ ТОМОГРАФИЯ

Макроскопически опухоль имеет дольчатое строение с наличием фиб-розных перегородок и центрального рубца, который, в отличие от очаговой узловой гиперплазии, является истинным. Размеры опухоли варьируют от 5 до 20 см. Хотя кровотечения встречаются редко, в 20–60% случаев отмечаются некроз и обызвествления, особенно в зоне центрального рубца. Чаще опухоль представляет собой солидное образование, хотя иногда наблюдается двудольчатость или же наличие сателлитов. Образование располагается внутри печени, хотя отмечены случаи опухоли «на ножке».

Микроскопическая картина фиброламеллярного рака характерна: эозинофильные злокачественные гепатоциты с четкими ядрами. Фиброзный компонент составляет до 50% массы опухоли и распространяется мультиламеллярными полосками, за исключением опухолей, содержащих крупные центральные рубцы. Часто имеются дополнительные узелки.

Клиническая картина весьма разнообразна. Чаще всего больные жалуются на боль, гепатомегалию, пальпируемое образование в правом верхнем квадранте брюшной полости и кахексию. Обычно на момент выявления опухоль достигает размеров более 15 см. Реже заболевание сопровождается болью, лихорадкой, симулирующей абсцесс печени, гинекомастией у мужчин, венозным тромбозом и желтухой. Гинекомастия является следствием превращения андрогенов в эстрогены при помощи фермента ароматазы, вырабатываемого злокачественными гепатоцитами.

Венозный тромбоз возникает вследствие инвазии опухоли в венозные

b)

Figure 4.6a,b. a - Page 25 from the book [4], section Fibrolamellar Carcinoma; b - Pages 450-451 from the book [1], section Fibrolamellar Carcinoma.

References

[1] Trufanov GE, Fokin BA (eds.) Magnetic Resonance Tomography. *Handbook for Physicians* (Russian). St. Petersburg: Foliant, 2007.

[2] EMRF Online http://www.emrf.org/New%20Site/FAQs/FAQs%20History%20of%20MRI.htm (accessed 26 June 2015).

[3] Bogaert J, Dymarkovski S, Taylor AM. (eds.) *Clinical Cardiac MRI.* Springer, 2005.

[4] Schneider G, Grazioli L, Saini S. (eds.) *MRI of the Liver: Technical Approach, Contrast-Enhanced Imaging, Differential Diagnosis*. 2nd edition. Springer, 2006.

Chapter 5

PLAGIARISM AND MISQUOTING IN ENVIRONMENTAL SCIENCE

SUMMARY

Environmental pathology is an increasingly important field of research because of the overpopulation and environmental pollution. These issues are of great public concern and need a responsible attitude. Nevertheless, misquoting, and misinterpretation of statistical data can be found in professional literature on environmental pathology from the former Soviet Union.

After the Chernobyl accident, many publications overestimated its medical consequences. Among the reasons were the heated interest in the Chernobyl topic that facilitated foreign help and international scientific cooperation. Moreover, the 'Chernobyl hysteria' has hindered advancement of nuclear power production in many countries, thus contributing to higher prices for fossil fuels. The following tools have been used for this purpose: interpretation of spontaneous diseases as radiation-induced, indication of radioactivity or dose levels without correlation with natural background radiation, conclusions about morbidity increase without statistically correct comparison with other regions, misquoting and misinterpretation of statistical data. Details and references are in Chapter 12.

INTRODUCTION

Environmental pathology is a field of increasing importance in our time of overpopulation and environmental pollution. These issues are of great public concern and, therefore, adherence to the generally accepted principles of research and publication is of particular importance. Unfortunately, misinterpretation of statistical data, plagiarism and misquoting can be found in professional literature on environmental pathology. Here are presented several examples.

THE EVIDENCE

Figure 5.1a is a photograph from page 103 of the article [1]. The borrowed text reads as follows: "For ^{131}I diagnostic procedures the dose rate decreases to 50% of its maximal value in about 6-7 days (with reduction to 1% of the maximal dose rate by about 50 days), in contrast to an exposure time of seconds or minutes for external exposure from an atomic bomb or radiotherapy" [1]. The corresponding paragraph from p. 26 of the Russian edition [2] shown in Figure 5.1b is translated as follows: "After an injection of ^{131}I, the radiation load on the thyroid increases gradually, attaining a maximum approximately one day after an injection of the radionuclide. The radiation dose to the thyroid decreases to 50% of its maximal level in 6-7 days and after that, in the course of about 50 days, decreases gradually to a 1% level. This is incomparable with several minutes, during which the thyroid is irradiated from external sources."

A mistranslation in the second sentence of the borrowed text caused an alteration of the meaning: the "dose rate" was mistranslated as the "radiation dose." In fact, it is the dose rate that is decreasing with time, while the dose itself continues accumulating. No reference to the source was given.

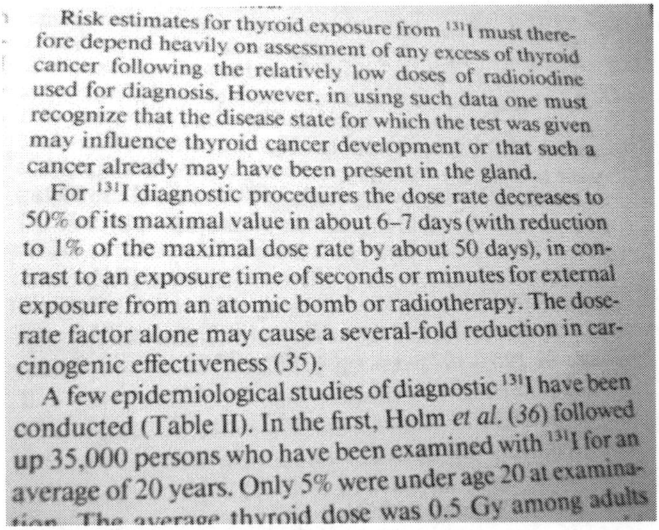

Risk estimates for thyroid exposure from ^{131}I must therefore depend heavily on assessment of any excess of thyroid cancer following the relatively low doses of radioiodine used for diagnosis. However, in using such data one must recognize that the disease state for which the test was given may influence thyroid cancer development or that such a cancer already may have been present in the gland.

For ^{131}I diagnostic procedures the dose rate decreases to 50% of its maximal value in about 6–7 days (with reduction to 1% of the maximal dose rate by about 50 days), in contrast to an exposure time of seconds or minutes for external exposure from an atomic bomb or radiotherapy. The dose-rate factor alone may cause a several-fold reduction in carcinogenic effectiveness (35).

A few epidemiological studies of diagnostic ^{131}I have been conducted (Table II). In the first, Holm *et al.* (36) followed up 35,000 persons who have been examined with ^{131}I for an average of 20 years. Only 5% were under age 20 at examination. The average thyroid dose was 0.5 Gy among adults

a)

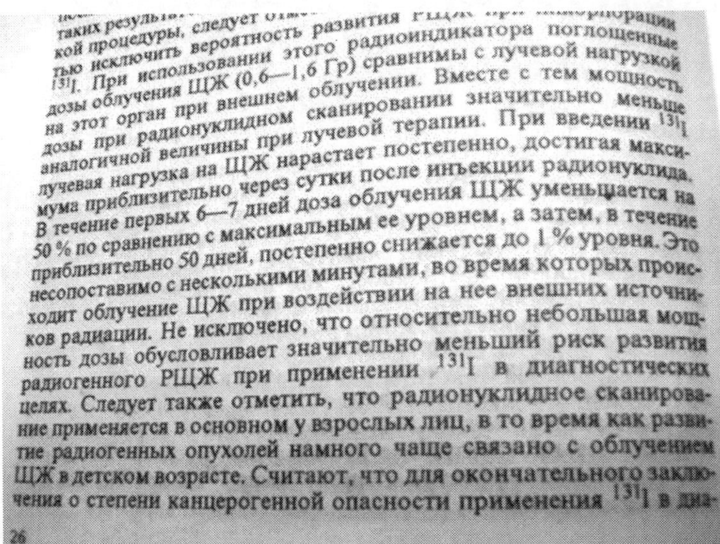

таких результатов, следует отметить … развития РЩЖ при инкорпорации
кой процедуры, вероятность радиоиндикатора поглощенные
тью исключить использовании этого сравнимы с лучевой нагрузкой
^{131}I. При облучения ЩЖ (0,6—1,6 Гр) облучении. Вместе с тем мощность
дозы облучения при внешнем сканировании значительно меньше
на этот орган при радионуклидном терапии. При введении ^{131}I
дозы при величины при лучевой постепенно, достигая макси-
аналогичной нагрузка на ЩЖ нарастает после инъекции радионуклида.
лучевая приблизительно через сутки облучения ЩЖ уменьшается на
мума первых 6—7 дней доза ее уровнем, а затем, в течение
В течение сравнению с максимальным снижается до 1 % уровня. Это
50 % по приблизительно 50 дней, постепенно во время которых проис-
несопоставимо с несколькими минутами, на нее внешних источни-
ходит облучение ЩЖ при воздействии относительно небольшая мощ-
ков радиации. Не исключено, что меньший риск развития
ность дозы обусловливает значительно ^{131}I в диагностических
радиогенного РЩЖ при применении
целях. Следует также отметить, что радионуклидное сканирова-
ние применяется в основном у взрослых лиц, в то время как разви-
тие радиогенных опухолей намного чаще связано с облучением
ЩЖ в детском возрасте. Считают, что для окончательного заклю-
чения о степени канцерогенной опасности применения ^{131}I в диа-

26

b)

Figure 5.1a,b. a - from p. 103 of the article [1]; b - Passage in the book [2] was borrowed from the 2nd paragraph in [1]. The borrowed text was found in the bottom paragraph on the page 26 [2].

Many publications that appeared after the Chernobyl accident overestimates medical consequences of the catastrophe. The overestimation went along with the overdiagnosis and overtreatment of certain diseases. In the first phase, heated interest in the Chernobyl incident facilitated foreign help and international scientific cooperation. Later, other motives became apparent: puffing up Chernobyl hysteria has hindered advancement of nuclear power production in many countries, thus boosting the prices for oil and gas [3, 4]. Examples can be found in publications [5-7].

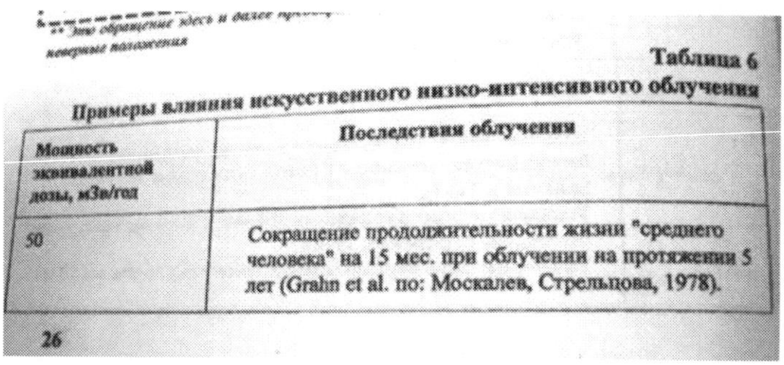
Таблица 6

Примеры влияния искусственного низко-интенсивного облучения

Мощность эквивалентной дозы, мЗв/год	Последствия облучения
50	Сокращение продолжительности жизни "среднего человека" на 15 мес. при облучении на протяжении 5 лет (Grahn et al. по: Москалев, Стрельцова, 1978).

26

Figure 5.2. A copy from page 26 of the book [6]. Translation: “Table 6. Equivalent dose rate 50 mSv/year. Consequences of radiation: Reduction of the life duration of an “average human” by 15 months after irradiation during 5 years (Grahn et al. after Moskalev, Streltsova, 1978).”

A corresponding publication by Moskalev and Streltsova from the year 1978 does not exist, which means that the publication year was printed wrong in the text (Figure 5.2), but correctly in the reference list of of the book [5] (Figure 5.4). The translation of the bottom paragraph from Figure 5.3 reads as follows: “According to the calculations by D. Grahn, G.A. Sacher, R.A. Lea et al. [270], the radiation dose of 2,5 Sv (i.e., 0,05 Sv yearly, obtained during 50 years of work, which is today the upper limit for occupational workers), received as chronic radiation during a very long time, can cause reduction of life duration by 15 days for an average 100-day-old mouse and approximately by 15 months for an average 20-year-old human.” This passage was misquoted in the book [6]. The key figure was changed from 50 to 5 years, thus creating an exaggerated impression about consequences of the exposure to low doses of ionizing radiation.

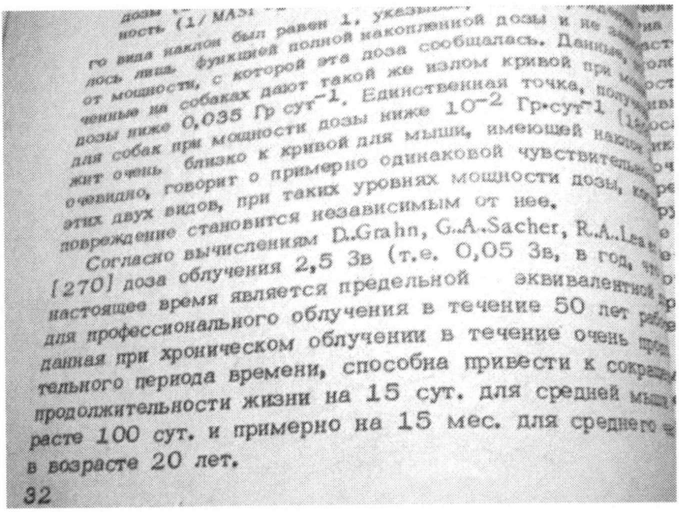

ность (1/ MA3I
го вида наклон был равен 1, указыв
лось лишь функцией полной накопленной дозы и не
от мощности, с которой эта доза сообщалась. Данные
ченные на собаках дают такой же излом кривой при
дозы ниже 0,035 Гр сут$^{-1}$. Единственная точка, получ
для собак при мощности дозы ниже 10^{-2} Гр·сут$^{-1}$
жит очень близко к кривой для мыши, имеющей
очевидно, говорит о примерно одинаковой чувствите
этих двух видов, при таких уровнях мощности дозы,
повреждение становится независимым от нее.
Согласно вычислениям D.Grahn, G.A.Sacher, R.A.L
[270] доза облучения 2,5 Зв (т.е. 0,05 Зв, в год,
настоящее время является предельной эквивалент
для профессионального облучения в течение 50 лет
данная при хроническом облучении в течение очень
тельного периода времени, способна привести к сокра
продолжительности жизни на 15 сут. для средней
расте 100 сут. и примерно на 15 мес. для среднего
в возрасте 20 лет.
32

Figure 5.3. A photograph taken from page 32 of the book by Moskalev and Streltsova, 1987 [8].

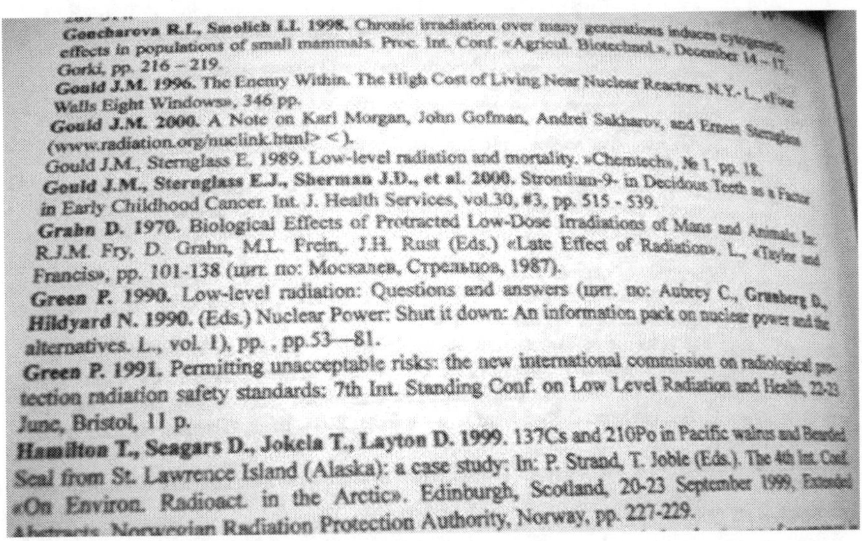

Goncharova R.I., Smolich I.I. 1998. Chronic irradiation over many generations induces cytogenetic effects in populations of small mammals. Proc. Int. Conf. «Agricul. Biotechnol.», December 14 – 17, Gorki, pp. 216 – 219.
Gould J.M. 1996. The Enemy Within. The High Cost of Living Near Nuclear Reactors. N.Y.- L., «Four Walls Eight Windows», 346 pp.
Gould J.M. 2000. A Note on Karl Morgan, John Gofman, Andrei Sakharov, and Ernest Sternglass (www.radiation.org/nuclink.html> <).
Gould J.M., Sternglass E. 1989. Low-level radiation and mortality. »Chemtech», № 1, pp. 18.
Gould J.M., Sternglass E.J., Sherman J.D., et al. 2000. Strontium-9- in Decidous Teeth as a Factor in Early Childhood Cancer. Int. J. Health Services, vol.30, #3, pp. 515 - 539.
Grahn D. 1970. Biological Effects of Protracted Low-Dose Irradiations of Mans and Animals. In: R.J.M. Fry, D. Grahn, M.L. Frein,. J.H. Rust (Eds.) «Late Effect of Radiation». L., «Taylor and Francis», pp. 101-138 (цит. по: Москалев, Стрельцов, 1987).
Green P. 1990. Low-level radiation: Questions and answers (цит. по: Aubrey C., Granberg D., **Hildyard N. 1990.** (Eds.) Nuclear Power: Shut it down: An information pack on nuclear power and the alternatives. L., vol. 1), pp. , pp.53—81.
Green P. 1991. Permitting unacceptable risks: the new international commission on radiological protection radiation safety standards: 7th Int. Standing Conf. on Low Level Radiation and Health, 22-23 June, Bristol, 11 p.
Hamilton T., Seagars D., Jokela T., Layton D. 1999. 137Cs and 210Po in Pacific walrus and Bearded Seal from St. Lawrence Island (Alaska): a case study: In: P. Strand, T. Joble (Eds.). The 4th Int. Conf. «On Environ. Radioact. in the Arctic». Edinburgh, Scotland, 20-23 September 1999, Extended Abstracts. Norwegian Radiation Protection Authority, Norway, pp. 227-229.

Figure 5.4. A photograph from the reference list of Yablokov [6]. The publication by Grahn et al. (1970) is quoted indirectly, after the publication referenced as Moskalev, Streltsova, 1987 [8].

The article by D. Grahn et al. from the year 1970 [9], the bibliographic description of which is similar (but not identical) to that presented in the reference list of the work by Yablokov [6] (Figure 5.4), was not quoted in [8] and, most importantly, it contains no passages similar to the cited above, which is in fact misquoting.

A publication with a corresponding passage, dated 1978 [10], was found according to the reference No. 270 (Figure 5.3) in the work by Moskalev and Streltsova [8]. Figure 5.5 shows the original text by D. Grahn et al. (1978): "A total dose of 250 rads delivered over the lifetime would produce 2.22% life shortening according to the data given here. This is 15 days for the average 100-day-old mouse and 445 days for the average 20-year-old human"; and further in the bottom paragraph: "Finally, the above example suggests that a total lifetime dose equal to the present maximum permissible dose of 5 rem per year for 50 years of occupational exposure, delivered at the rate of about 100 mrem per week, would induce a 15-month reduction of life expectancy" [10] (Figure 5.5).

approximately the same as the α term of 65 x 10^{-6}/R, given by Sacher [26] as the low dose-rate dose-effect constant for mice that was derived by a somewhat different approach [27,28].

A total dose of 250 rads delivered over the lifetime would produce 2.22% life shortening according to the data given here. This is 15 days for the average 100-day-old mouse and 445 days for the average 20-year-old human. Life shortening for man would amount to about 1.8 days per rad, which is slightly greater than the figure of 1.2 days derived on the basis of the relation between MAS and the daily exposure level. The comparison of these values does not involve a truly independent pair of estimates, however, because the same data contribute to both. Different analytical pathways are used, though they eventually converge on the assumption that man:mouse extrapolation relies upon the ratio of life table constants.

Finally, the above example suggests that a total lifetime dose equal to the present maximum permissible dose of 5 rem per year for 50 years of occupational exposure, delivered at the rate of about 100 mrem per week, would induce a 15-month reduction in life expectancy.

Figure 5.5. Text from p. 57 of the article [10].

This paragraph is misquoted in [8]: the unit of absorbed radiation dose "rad" was replaced by the equivalent dose unit "Sievert" (which is not the same), whereas the "lifetime" was replaced by "very long time."

In sum, the text fragment from [10], incorrectly quoted by Moskalev and Streltsova in 1987 [8] was then further misquoted by Yablokov in 2002 [6], who cited it indirectly after [8]. This example demonstrates how the "second-hand" citation can lead a distortion of the original information.

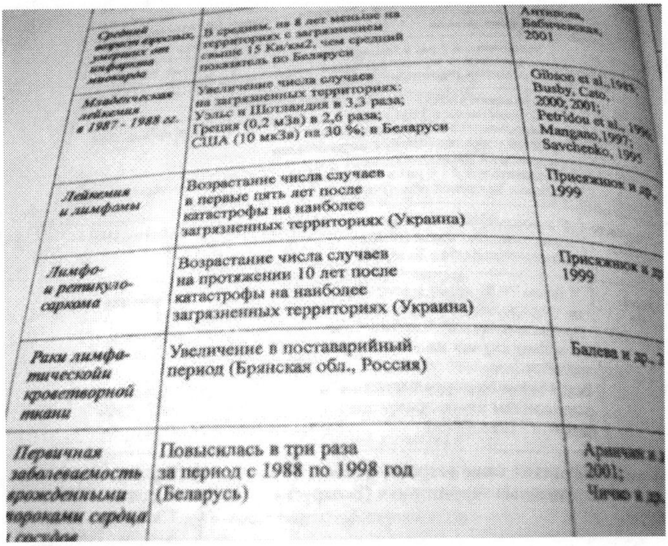

Средний возраст взрослых умерших от инфарктов миокарда	В среднем, на 8 лет меньше на территориях с загрязнением свыше 15 Ки/км2, чем средний показатель по Беларуси	Антипова, Бабиченко, 2001
Младенческая лейкемия в 1987 - 1988 гг.	Увеличение числа случаев на загрязненных территориях: Уэльс и Шотландия в 3,3 раза; Греция (0,2 мЗв) в 2,6 раза; США (10 мкЗв) на 30 %; в Беларуси	Gibson et al., 1988; Busby, Cato, 2000; 2001; Petridou et al., 1996; Mangano, 1997; Savchenko, 1995
Лейкемии и лимфомы	Возрастание числа случаев в первые пять лет после катастрофы на наиболее загрязненных территориях (Украина)	Присяжнюк и др., 1999
Лимфо- и ретикуло-саркома	Возрастание числа случаев на протяжении 10 лет после катастрофы на наиболее загрязненных территориях (Украина)	Присяжнюк и др., 1999
Раки лимфатической кроветворной ткани	Увеличение в поставарийный период (Брянская обл., Россия)	Балева и др., 2
Первичная заболеваемость врожденными пороками сердца и сосудов	Повысилась в три раза за период с 1988 по 1998 год (Беларусь)	Аракчян и [illegible] 2001; Чичко и др.

Figure 5.6. A table from the book [6].

The table (Figure 5.6) contains information about medical consequences of the Chernobyl accident with corresponding references. The data about morbidity increase after the accident are not in agreement with the UNSCEAR (2000) report, according to which, apart from the thyroid cancer increase in children and adolescents, there was no evidence of any major public health impact attributable to radiation exposure after the Chernobyl accident [11]. Most remarkable is the second line of the table, where the British Islands, Greece, and the United States are listed among territories contaminated with radionuclides after the Chernobyl accident. Translation of the second line of the table in Figure 5.6 reads: "Leukemia in infants 1987-1988. Increase of the number of cases in contaminated territories: Wales and Scotland 3.3 times; Greece (0,2 mSv) 2,6 times; U.S.A. (10 mkSv) by 30% (Gibson et al., 1988; Busby, Cato 2000, 2001; Petridou et al., 1996; Mangano 1997; Savchenko 1995)" [6].

CHILDHOOD LEUKAEMIA REGISTRATIONS IN SCOTLAND 1971–87

	1971–80		1981–86		1987	
Age (yr)	Observed	Annual*	Observed	Expected	Observed	Expected†
0	15	2·1	9	7·7	6	1·4
1–4	201	6·7	105	104·0	27	17·2
5–9	131	3·0	51	57·7	7	9·4
10–14	91	2·0	33	46·7	8	6·9
Total	438	. .	198	216·1	48	34·9

*Rate/10^6. †Calculated on basis of 1986 populations.

Figure 5.7. A table from [12].

The statement about 3.3-fold increase in the incidence of childhood leukemia in Wales and Scotland in the years 1987-1988 can be related only to the first line of the table containing the following figures: 1971-1980 (15 cases); 1981-1986 (9 cases) and the year 1987 (6 cases) [12] (Figure 5.6). Gibson et al. (1988) did not put these figures in connection with the Chernobyl accident. The whole body scanning for radiocaesium performed by Gibson et al. in some of the children and their mothers did not demonstrate any increased levels compared to controls [12]. Moreover, one year is too short for induction of radiogenic leukemia [13]. Overall, this example should be qualified as misinterpretation of published data.

The publication by Yablokov, best known in the West, is titled "Radioactive waste disposal in seas adjacent to the territory of the Russian Federation" [5]. It extracts materials from the report of a Commission prepared in Russia in 1993. The Commission submitted the report to the President of the Russian Federation in February 1993. By Presidential decision, this report (after several technical corrections) was available to the public: it is known as "the Yablokov Commission report" or simply the "Yablokov Report." During April-May 1993, 500 copies were distributed among governmental agencies inside Russia and abroad through a net of Russian Embassies (Editor's note to [5]). The article [5] has no references and no clear conclusions, the most significant numerical value being 325 kCi, which is the estimated total activity of wastes dumped in seas adjacent to the Russian territory (contamination due to the nuclear testing was not discussed). A possible upper limit of this value was supposed as high as

2.5 MCi [5]. Only the latter figure, not corroborated in the text of the article, is given in the open access abstract [5], which can be classified as a misrepresentation of numerical data.

CONCLUSION

The plagiarism, misquoting and data manipulation can be found in the professional literature on environmental pathology from the former Soviet Union in spite of the considerable public concern and responsibility associated with this topic. False or tendentious citations were used for the purpose of overestimation of medical consequences of the Chernobyl accident thereby fostering radiophobia. It has become clear today that "Chernobyl hysteria" has hindered advancement of nuclear power production in many countries, thus contributing to higher prices for fossil fuels, of which more in Chapter 12.

REFERENCES

[1] Shore RE. Issues and epidemiological evidence regarding radiation-induced thyroid cancer. *Radiat Res* 1992;131(1):98-111.

[2] Demidchik EP, Tsyb AF, Lushnikov EF. *Rak shitovidnoi zhelezy u detei. Posledstviya avarii na Chernobylskoi AES* [*Thyroid carcinoma in children. Consequences of the accident at Chernobyl power station*]. Moscow: Meditsina, 1996.

[3] Jargin SV. *The Overestimation of Medical Consequences of Low-Dose Exposure to Ionizing Radiation.* Newcastle upon Tyne: Cambridge Scholars Publishing, 2019.

[4] Jargin SV. Overestimation of Chernobyl consequences: biophysical aspects. *Radiat Environ Biophys* 2009;48(3):341-4.

[5] Yablokov AV. Radioactive waste disposal in seas adjacent to the territory of the Russian Federation. *Mar Pollut Bull* 2001;43(1-6):8-18.

[6] Yablokov AV. *Mif o bezopasnosti malych doz radiatsii* [*A mythos about safety of small radiation doses*] Moscow: Center for Russian Environmental Policy, 2002.

[7] Yablokov AV. Consequences of Chernobyl catastrophe for public health: criticism of the IAEA/WHO position (in Russian). *Report at the Congress* [*Problems of radiation biology and human safety*] (July 3, 2008, Saint-Petersburg, http://ecoforum2008.com/en/preliminary/rad/). An abstract (in Russian) is published in: Vestnik Rossiiskoi voenno-meditsinskoiakademii. 2008;23(3) Suppl 2(Part 1):241-2.

[8] Moskalev IuI., Streltsova VN. Otdalennye posledstviya radiatsionnogo porazheniya. Neopukholevye formy [Late consequences of radiation damage. Non-tumorous forms] *Series "Radiatsionnaya biologiya"* [*Radiation biology*] Vol. 6. Moscow: VINITI, 1987; p. 32.

[9] Grahn D. Biological effects of protracted low dose radiation exposure of man and animals. In: *Late Effects of Radiation* (R. J. M. Fry, D. Grahn, M. L. Griem and J. H. Rust, Eds.), London: Taylor & Francis, 1970; pp. 101-136.

[10] Grahn D., Sacher GA, Lea RA, Fry RJM, Rust JH. Analytical approaches to and interpretation of data on time, rate and cause of death of mice exposed to external gamma irradiation. In: *Late Biological Effects of Ionizing Radiation.* Vienna: IAEA, 1978; pp. 43-58.

[11] UNSCEAR 2000 Report to the General Assembly. Vol. 1. *Sources and effects of ionizing radiation.* New York: United Nations, 2000.

[12] Gibson BE. Eden OB, Barrett A, Stiller CA, Draper GJ. Leukemia in young children in Scotland. *Lancet* 1988;2(8611):630.

[13] Ron E. Ionizing radiation and cancer risk: evidence from epidemiology. *Radiat Res* 1998;150(5 Suppl):S30-41.

Chapter 6

HISTORICAL EXAMPLES

INTRODUCTION

Here we are presenting several examples of plagiarism and misquoting from the history of pathology. The source of borrowings in all examples presented here was the Handbuch der Speziellen Pathologischen Anatomie und Histologie edited by Friedrich Henke and Otto Lubarsch, published by Julius Springer in Berlin (volume 4 part 2 edited in1928 and volume 6 part 1 edited in 1930) [1-3]. The borrowings were found in the chapter on pathology of the stomach, written by Yuli Lazovski and in the chapter on pathology of the liver, written by Alexey Abrikosov, in the Handbook of Pathological Anatomy in Many Volumes (editor: A.I. Strukov; editor of the volume on pathology of the digestive organs A.I. Abrikosov), published by Medgiz in Moscow in 1957 [4, 5].

Example 1

The text in German on the stomach lesions in congenital syphilis on pages 1017-1018 of volume 4, part 2 in Handbuch der Speziellen

Pathologischen Anatomie und Histologie [1] (Figure 6.1a,b) reads as follows:

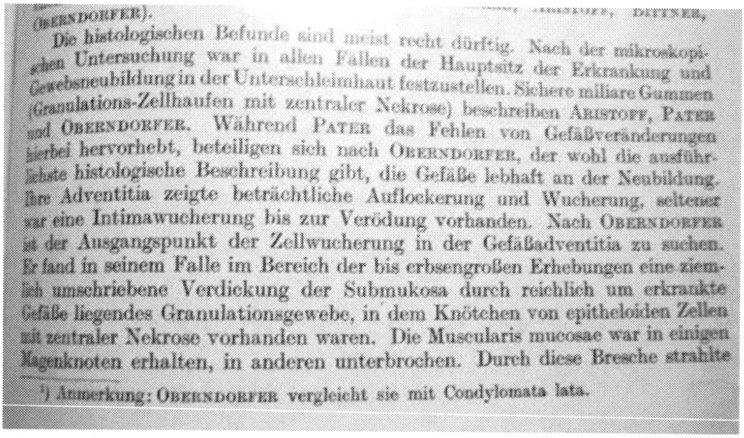

(Oberndorfer).

Die histologischen Befunde sind meist recht dürftig. Nach der mikroskopischen Untersuchung war in allen Fällen der Hauptsitz der Erkrankung und Gewebsneubildung in der Unterschleimhaut festzustellen. Sichere miliare Gummen (Granulations-Zellhaufen mit zentraler Nekrose) beschreiben Aristoff, Pater und Oberndorfer. Während Pater das Fehlen von Gefäßveränderungen hierbei hervorhebt, beteiligen sich nach Oberndorfer, der wohl die ausführlichste histologische Beschreibung gibt, die Gefäße lebhaft an der Neubildung. Ihre Adventitia zeigte beträchtliche Auflockerung und Wucherung, seltener war eine Intimawucherung bis zur Verödung vorhanden. Nach Oberndorfer ist der Ausgangspunkt der Zellwucherung in der Gefäßadventitia zu suchen. Er fand in seinem Falle im Bereich der bis erbsengroßen Erhebungen eine ziemlich umschriebene Verdickung der Submukosa durch reichlich um erkrankte Gefäße liegendes Granulationsgewebe, in dem Knötchen von epitheloiden Zellen mit zentraler Nekrose vorhanden waren. Die Muscularis mucosae war in einigen Magenknoten erhalten, in anderen unterbrochen. Durch diese Bresche strahlte

[1]) Anmerkung: Oberndorfer vergleicht sie mit Condylomata lata.

a)

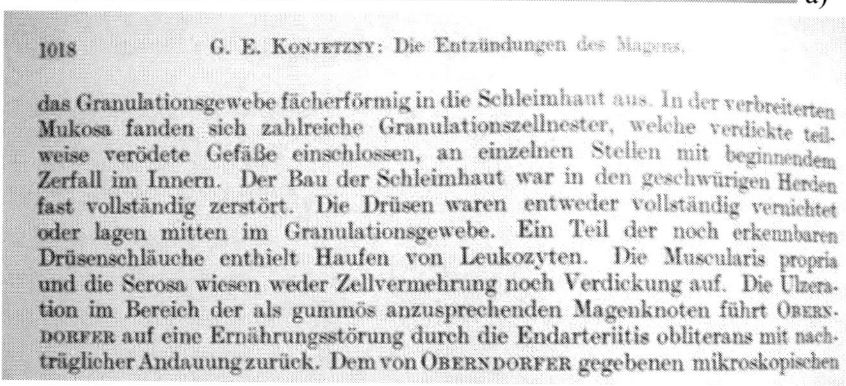

1018 G. E. Konjetzny: Die Entzündungen des Magens.

das Granulationsgewebe fächerförmig in die Schleimhaut aus. In der verbreiterten Mukosa fanden sich zahlreiche Granulationszellnester, welche verdickte teilweise verödete Gefäße einschlossen, an einzelnen Stellen mit beginnendem Zerfall im Innern. Der Bau der Schleimhaut war in den geschwürigen Herden fast vollständig zerstört. Die Drüsen waren entweder vollständig vernichtet oder lagen mitten im Granulationsgewebe. Ein Teil der noch erkennbaren Drüsenschläuche enthielt Haufen von Leukozyten. Die Muscularis propria und die Serosa wiesen weder Zellvermehrung noch Verdickung auf. Die Ulzeration im Bereich der als gummös anzusprechenden Magenknoten führt Oberndorfer auf eine Ernährungsstörung durch die Endarteriitis obliterans mit nachträglicher Andauung zurück. Dem von Oberndorfer gegebenen mikroskopischen

b)

Figure 6.1a,b. Stomach lesions in congenital syphilis. Reproduced from Handbuch der Speziellen Pathologischen Anatomie und Histologie, 1928 [1].

"Nach der mikroskopischen Untersuchung war in allen Fällen der Hauptsitz der Erkrankung und Gewebsneubildung in der Unterschleimhaut festzustellen. Sichere miliare Gummen (Granulations-Zellhaufen mit zentraler Nekrose) beschrieben Aristoff, Pater und Oberndorfer. Während Pater das Fehlen von Gefäßveränderungen hierbei hervorhebt, beteiligen sich nach Oberndorfer, der wohl die ausführlichste histologische Beschreibung gibt, die Gefäße lebhaft an der Neubildung. Ihre Adventitia zeigte beträchtliche Auflockerung und Wucherung, seltener war eine Intimawucherung bis zur Verödung vorhanden. Nach

Oberndorfer ist der Ausgangspunkt der Zellwucherung in der Gefäßadventitia zu suchen. Er fand in seinem Falle im Bereich der bis erbsengroßen Erhebungen eine ziemlich umschriebene Verdickung der Submucosa durch reichlich um erkrankte Gefäße liegendes Granulationsgewebe, in dem Knötchen von epitheloiden Zellen mit zentraler Nekrose vorhanden waren. Die Muscularis mucosae war in einigen Magenknoten erhalten, in anderen unterbrochen. Durch diese Bresche strahlte das Granulationsgewebe in die Schleimhaut aus. In der verbreiterten Mucosa fanden sich zahlreiche Granulationszellnester, welche verdickte teilweise verödete Gefäße einschlossen, an einzelnen Stellen mit beginnendem Zerfall im Inneren. Der Bau der Schleimhaut war in den geschwürigen Herden fast vollständig zerstört… Die Muscularis propria und die Serosa wiesen weder Zellvermehrung noch Verdickung auf" [1].

This text can be translated into English as follows:

"Microscopically, the main location of the pathological changes and of the newly formed tissue in all cases was the submucosa. Unequivocal miliary gummas (collections of granuloma cells with central necrosis) were described by Aristoff, Pater and Oberndorfer. Pater pointed out the absence of vascular changes; but according to Oberndorfer (who provided probably the most detailed histological description) blood vessels vividly participate on the new formation. The adventitia showed considerable loosening and excrescence but the overgrowth of the intima up to the lumen obsolescence was rarer. According to Oberndorfer, the starting point of cellular proliferation must be searched within the vascular adventitia. He found in his case, in the area of up to pea-sized elevations, a rather well delimited thickening of the submucosa caused by abundant granulation tissue formed around pathologically changed blood vessels. Nodules of epithelioid cells with central necrosis were present in the granulation tissue. The muscularis mucosae was preserved in some gastric nodules, but interrupted in other ones. Granulation tissue radiated through these breaches into the mucosa. In the widened mucosa, numerous foci of granulation cells were found around thickened and partly obsolete blood vessels, in some places with beginning decomposition inside. The structure of the mucosa was almost completely destroyed within the foci of ulceration… The muscularis propria and serosa showed neither increased cellulation nor thickening" [1].

The text by Lazovski from page 390 of the handbook [4] is shown in Figure 6.2. It can be translated as follows:

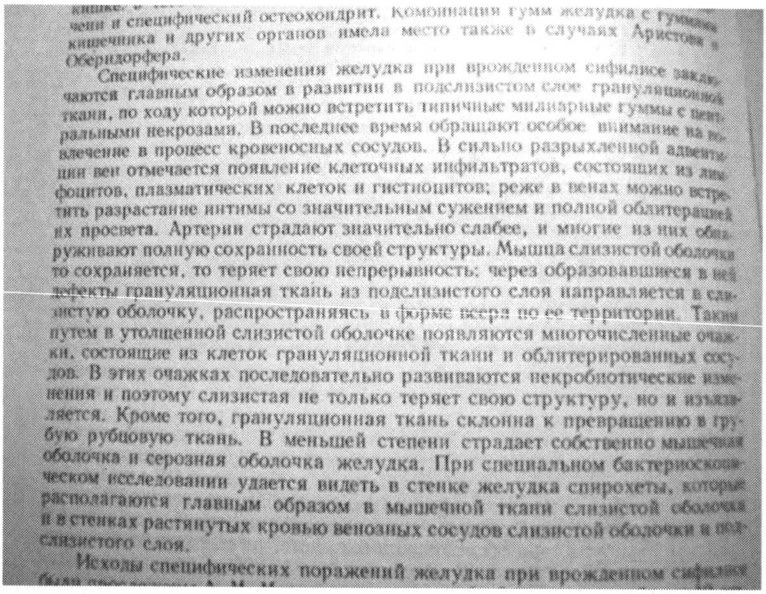
чени и специфический остеохондрит. Комбинация гумм желудка с гуммами кишечника и других органов имела место также в случаях Аристова и Оберндорфера.

Специфические изменения желудка при врожденном сифилисе заключаются главным образом в развитии в подслизистом слое грануляционной ткани, по ходу которой можно встретить типичные милиарные гуммы с центральными некрозами. В последнее время обращают особое внимание на вовлечение в процесс кровеносных сосудов. В сильно разрыхленной адвентиции вен отмечается появление клеточных инфильтратов, состоящих из лимфоцитов, плазматических клеток и гистиоцитов; реже в венах можно встретить разрастание интимы со значительным сужением и полной облитерацией их просвета. Артерии страдают значительно слабее, и многие из них обнаруживают полную сохранность своей структуры. Мышца слизистой оболочки то сохраняется, то теряет свою непрерывность; через образовавшиеся в ней дефекты грануляционная ткань из подслизистого слоя направляется в слизистую оболочку, распространяясь в форме веера по ее территории. Таким путем в утолщенной слизистой оболочке появляются многочисленные очажки, состоящие из клеток грануляционной ткани и облитерированных сосудов. В этих очажках последовательно развиваются некробиотические изменения и поэтому слизистая не только теряет свою структуру, но и изъязвляется. Кроме того, грануляционная ткань склонна к превращению в грубую рубцовую ткань. В меньшей степени страдает собственно мышечная оболочка и серозная оболочка желудка. При специальном бактериоскопическом исследовании удается видеть в стенке желудка спирохеты, которые располагаются главным образом в мышечной ткани слизистой оболочки и в стенках растянутых кровью венозных сосудов слизистой оболочки и подслизистого слоя.

Исходы специфических поражений желудка при врожденном сифилисе

Figure 6.2. Stomach lesions in congenital syphilis. Reproduced from the Mnogotomnoe rukovodstvo po patologicheskoi anatomii [Handbook of pathological anatomy in many volumes], 1957 [4].

"Specific gastric changes in congenital syphilis are mainly represented by development of granulation tissue in the submucosa, where typical miliary gummas with central necrosis can be found. Last time, special attention has been drawn to the involvement of blood vessels into the process. In the considerably loosened venous adventitia appear numerous cellular infiltrates composed of lymphocytes, plasma cells, and histiocytes; rarer is the overgrowth of the intima with a narrowing or obsolescence of the lumen... . The muscularis mucosae is preserved in some places, but interrupted in other ones. Granulation tissue radiates through these breaches into the mucosa. Thus in the widened mucosa appear numerous foci consisting of granulation tissue and obliterated vessels. In these foci, necrobiotic changes are consequently developing, and therefore structure of the mucosa is destroyed, and the mucosa becomes ulcerated. The gastric muscularis propria and serosa are less affected" [4].

Comment

The Russian text is shortened; but the flow of ideas is identical to the original. Interestingly, Iu.M. Lazovski, writing his work in the late 1950s on the basis of the handbook from the 1920s, expresses the G.E. Konjetzny's notion (based on the references to still earlier publications) about involvement of blood vessels in syphilis using the idiom "last time": "Last time, the attention has been drawn to the involvement of blood vessels into the process" [4].

Example 2

The text on the stomach ulcers and scars in syphilis on pages 1024-1025 of volume 4, part 2 of Handbuch der Speziellen Pathologischen Anatomie und Histologie [1] (Figure 6.3) reads as follows:

> "Einfache Ulzera und Narben
>
> Ganz ähnlich wie bei der chronischen Gastritis liegen die Dinge in den Fällen, in welchen bei Syphilitischen einfache typische chronische Ulzera und Narben im Magen gefunden worden sind. Bekanntlich hat ja Cruveilhier die Meinung ausgesprochen, daß wenigstens ein Teil der einfachen Magengeschwüre syphilitischen Ursprungs ist. Auch Galliard glaubt, daß viele Ulcera rotunda auf syphilitischer Grundlage (syphilitische Gefäßerkrankungen) entstehen. Nach Lang sollen 29% aller Magengeschwüre auf Syphilitische entfallen. Diese Feststellung ist vielfach in dem Sinne bewertet worden, daß Magengeschwüre bei Syphilitischen besonders häufig sind. … Chiari hat unter seinen 97 Fällen von erworbener Syphilis … nur einmal ein einfaches Magengeschwür

und in dem gleichen Fall eine augenscheinlich auf ein solches Ulcus zu beziehende Narbe… "Der Magen syphilitischer Individuen ist gewiß nicht häufiger als der anderer Personen Sitz von peptischen Ulzerationen oder darauf zu beziehender Narben." [1]

This text can be translated as follows:

> "Simple ulcers and scars
>
> The issue of typical simple ulcers and scars in the stomach of a syphilitic patient is analogous to that of the chronic gastritis. Cruveilhier pointed out that at least a part of simple stomach ulcers are of syphilitic nature. Also Galliard believes that many round ulcers appear on the basis of syphilis (syphilitic vascular disease). According to Lang, 29% of all stomach ulcers must be found in syphilitics. This statement should be valued largely in the sense that stomach ulcers are especially frequent in syphilitic patients... . Chiari had among his 97 cases of acquired syphilis only 1 stomach ulcer and in the same case a scar obviously related to such an ulcer ... . 'The stomach of a syphilitic individual houses peptic ulcers or scars related to the ulcers certainly not more frequently than that of other persons'" [1].

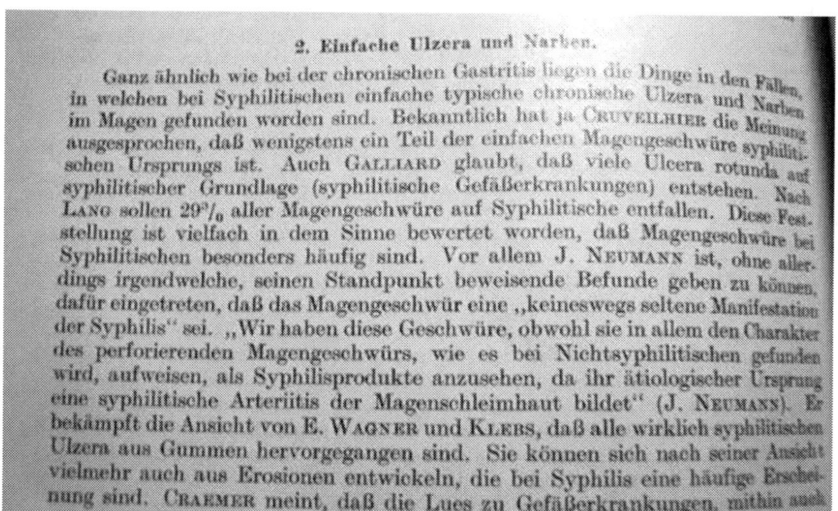

2. Einfache Ulzera und Narben.

Ganz ähnlich wie bei der chronischen Gastritis liegen die Dinge in den Fällen, in welchen bei Syphilitischen einfache typische chronische Ulzera und Narben im Magen gefunden worden sind. Bekanntlich hat ja CRUVEILHIER die Meinung ausgesprochen, daß wenigstens ein Teil der einfachen Magengeschwüre syphilitischen Ursprungs ist. Auch GALLIARD glaubt, daß viele Ulcera rotunda auf syphilitischer Grundlage (syphilitische Gefäßerkrankungen) entstehen. Nach LANG sollen 29% aller Magengeschwüre auf Syphilitische entfallen. Diese Feststellung ist vielfach in dem Sinne bewertet worden, daß Magengeschwüre bei Syphilitischen besonders häufig sind. Vor allem J. NEUMANN ist, ohne allerdings irgendwelche, seinen Standpunkt beweisende Befunde geben zu können, dafür eingetreten, daß das Magengeschwür eine „keineswegs seltene Manifestation der Syphilis" sei. „Wir haben diese Geschwüre, obwohl sie in allem den Charakter des perforierenden Magengeschwürs, wie es bei Nichtsyphilitischen gefunden wird, aufweisen, als Syphilisprodukte anzusehen, da ihr ätiologischer Ursprung eine syphilitische Arteriitis der Magenschleimhaut bildet" (J. NEUMANN). Er bekämpft die Ansicht von E. WAGNER und KLEBS, daß alle wirklich syphilitischen Ulzera aus Gummen hervorgegangen sind. Sie können sich nach seiner Ansicht vielmehr auch aus Erosionen entwickeln, die bei Syphilis eine häufige Erscheinung sind. CRAEMER meint, daß die Lues zu Gefäßerkrankungen, mithin auch

a)

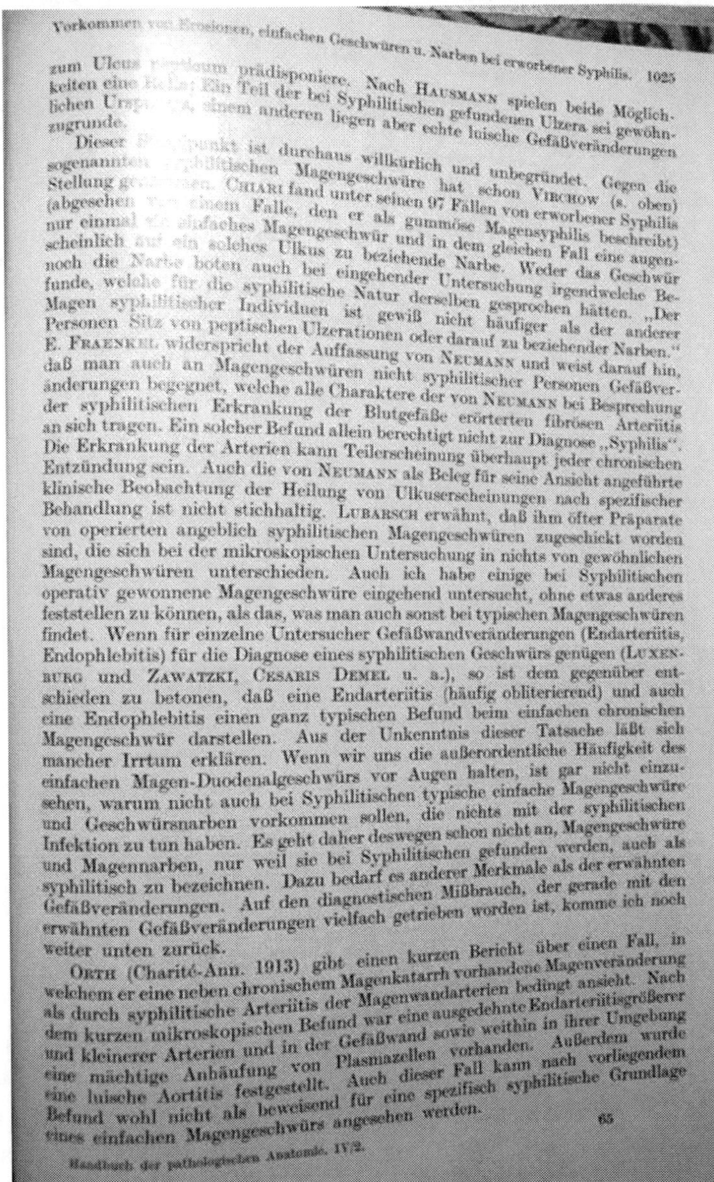
Vorkommen von Erosionen, einfachen Geschwüren u. Narben bei erworbener Syphilis. 1025

zum Ulcus [illegible] prädisponiere. Nach HAUSMANN spielen beide Möglich-
keiten eine Rolle: Ein Teil der bei Syphilitischen gefundenen Ulzera sei gewöhn-
lichen Ursprungs, einem anderen liegen aber echte luische Gefäßveränderungen
zugrunde.

Dieser Standpunkt ist durchaus willkürlich und unbegründet. Gegen die
sogenannten syphilitischen Magengeschwüre hat schon VIRCHOW (s. oben)
Stellung genommen. CHIARI fand unter seinen 97 Fällen von erworbener Syphilis
(abgesehen von einem Falle, den er als gummöse Magensyphilis beschreibt)
nur einmal ein einfaches Magengeschwür und in dem gleichen Fall eine augen-
scheinlich auf ein solches Ulkus zu beziehende Narbe. Weder das Geschwür
noch die Narbe boten auch bei eingehender Untersuchung irgendwelche Be-
funde, welche für die syphilitische Natur derselben gesprochen hätten. „Der
Magen syphilitischer Individuen ist gewiß nicht häufiger als der anderer
Personen Sitz von peptischen Ulzerationen oder darauf zu beziehender Narben."
E. FRAENKEL widerspricht der Auffassung von NEUMANN und weist darauf hin,
daß man auch an Magengeschwüren nicht syphilitischer Personen Gefäßver-
änderungen begegnet, welche alle Charaktere der von NEUMANN bei Besprechung
der syphilitischen Erkrankung der Blutgefäße erörterten fibrösen Arteriitis
an sich tragen. Ein solcher Befund allein berechtigt nicht zur Diagnose „Syphilis".
Die Erkrankung der Arterien kann Teilerscheinung überhaupt jeder chronischen
Entzündung sein. Auch die von NEUMANN als Beleg für seine Ansicht angeführte
klinische Beobachtung der Heilung von Ulkuserscheinungen nach spezifischer
Behandlung ist nicht stichhaltig. LUBARSCH erwähnt, daß ihm öfter Präparate
von operierten angeblich syphilitischen Magengeschwüren zugeschickt worden
sind, die sich bei der mikroskopischen Untersuchung in nichts von gewöhnlichen
Magengeschwüren unterschieden. Auch ich habe einige bei Syphilitischen
operativ gewonnene Magengeschwüre eingehend untersucht, ohne etwas anderes
feststellen zu können, als das, was man auch sonst bei typischen Magengeschwüren
findet. Wenn für einzelne Untersucher Gefäßwandveränderungen (Endarteriitis,
Endophlebitis) für die Diagnose eines syphilitischen Geschwürs genügen (LUXEN-
BURG und ZAWATZKI, CESARIS DEMEL u. a.), so ist dem gegenüber ent-
schieden zu betonen, daß eine Endarteriitis (häufig obliterierend) und auch
eine Endophlebitis einen ganz typischen Befund beim einfachen chronischen
Magengeschwür darstellen. Aus der Unkenntnis dieser Tatsache läßt sich
mancher Irrtum erklären. Wenn wir uns die außerordentliche Häufigkeit des
einfachen Magen-Duodenalgeschwürs vor Augen halten, ist gar nicht einzu-
sehen, warum nicht auch bei Syphilitischen typische einfache Magengeschwüre
und Geschwürsnarben vorkommen sollen, die nichts mit der syphilitischen
Infektion zu tun haben. Es geht daher deswegen schon nicht an, Magengeschwüre
und Magennarben, nur weil sie bei Syphilitischen gefunden werden, auch als
syphilitisch zu bezeichnen. Dazu bedarf es anderer Merkmale als der erwähnten
Gefäßveränderungen. Auf den diagnostischen Mißbrauch, der gerade mit den
erwähnten Gefäßveränderungen vielfach getrieben worden ist, komme ich noch
weiter unten zurück.

ORTH (Charité-Ann. 1913) gibt einen kurzen Bericht über einen Fall, in
welchem er eine neben chronischem Magenkatarrh vorhandene Magenveränderung
als durch syphilitische Arteriitis der Magenwandarterien bedingt ansieht. Nach
dem kurzen mikroskopischen Befund war eine ausgedehnte Endarteriitis größerer
und kleinerer Arterien und in der Gefäßwand sowie weithin in ihrer Umgebung
eine mächtige Anhäufung von Plasmazellen vorhanden. Außerdem wurde
eine luische Aortitis festgestellt. Auch dieser Fall kann nach vorliegendem
Befund wohl nicht als beweisend für eine spezifisch syphilitische Grundlage
eines einfachen Magengeschwürs angesehen werden.

Handbuch der pathologischen Anatomie. IV/2. 65

b)

Figure 6.3a,b. Stomach ulcers and scars in syphilis. Reproduced from Handbuch der Speziellen Pathologischen Anatomie und Histologie, 1928 [1].

Все функциональные заболевания желудка у больных сифилисом следует выделить в особую рубрику, как это совершенно правильно делает Р. А. Лурия, куда необходимо отнести, например, желудочные кризы у табетиков. Паль и Шлезингер идут еще дальше, утверждая, что у сифилитиков чаще наблюдаются функционально-нервные заболевания желудка, чем грубо анатомические. Что касается морфологического субстрата этих заболеваний, их патогенеза, отношения к подлинным воспалительным процессам и, наконец, принадлежности к сифилитической инфекции, то все эти вопросы остаются открытыми и требуют специального изучения.

2. Простые язвы и рубцы. Вопрос об их сифилитической природе обсуждается еще со времени Крювелье. Он впервые высказал мнение, что часть хронических язв желудка необходимо поставить в патогенетическую связь с сифилисом. Это мнение было поддержано в дальнейшем рядом авторов, которые с категоричностью утверждали, что хроническая язва желудка—далеко нередкое проявление сифилитической инфекции (по Лангу, 20% язв желудка имеют сифилогенное происхождение). После работы Хиари, установившего, что у больных сифилисом хронические язвы в желудке встречаются не более часто, чем у других больных, подобного

---

[1] В работе Эйстермана из 93 (!) приводимых случаев сифилиса желудка гистологическому обследованию подверглось только 10.

a)

...ке и специфический остеохондрит. Комбинации гумм желудка с гуммами кишечника и других органов имела место также в случаях Аристова и Обериндорфера.

Специфические изменения желудка при врожденном сифилисе заключаются главным образом в развитии в подслизистом слое грануляционной ткани, по ходу которой можно встретить типичные милиарные гуммы с центральными некрозами. В последнее время обращают особое внимание на вовлечение в процесс кровеносных сосудов. В сильно разрыхленной адвентиции вен отмечается появление клеточных инфильтратов, состоящих из лимфоцитов, плазматических клеток и гистиоцитов; реже в венах можно встретить разрастание интимы со значительным сужением и полной облитерацией их просвета. Артерии страдают значительно слабее, и многие из них обнаруживают полную сохранность своей структуры. Мышца слизистой оболочки то сохраняется, то теряет свою непрерывность: через образовавшиеся в ней дефекты грануляционная ткань из подслизистого слоя направляется в слизистую оболочку, распространяясь в форме веера по ее территории. Таким путем в утолщенной слизистой оболочке появляются многочисленные очажки, состоящие из клеток грануляционной ткани и облитерированных сосудов. В этих очажках последовательно развиваются некробиотические изменения и поэтому слизистая не только теряет свою структуру, но и изъязвляется. Кроме того, грануляционная ткань склонна к превращению в грубую рубцовую ткань. В меньшей степени страдает собственно мышечная оболочка и серозная оболочка желудка. При специальном бактериоскопическом исследовании удается видеть в стенке желудка спирохеты, которые располагаются главным образом в мышечной ткани слизистой оболочки и в стенках растянутых кровью венозных сосудов слизистой оболочки и подслизистого слоя.

Исходы специфических поражений желудка при врожденном сифилисе ...

b)

Figure 6.4a,b. Stomach ulcers and scars in syphilis. Reproduced from Mnogotomnoe rukovodstvo po patologicheskoi anatomii [Handbook of pathological anatomy in many volumes], 1957 [4].

The text by Lazovski from the pages 391-392 of the handbook [4] is shown in Figure 6.4a,b. It can be translated as follows:

> "Simple ulcers and scars
>
> The issue of their syphilitic nature is discussed since the time of Cruveilhier. He first pointed out that a part of chronic stomach ulcers should be put in connection with syphilis.
>
> This opinion was later supported by some authors, who stated categorically that a chronic gastric ulcer is a frequent expression of the syphilitic infection (according to Lang, 20% of all stomach ulcers are of syphilogenic origin).
>
> After the Chiari's work, who determined that chronic stomach ulcers in syphilitics are not more frequent than in other patients, such statements started already to acquire historical interest" [4].

Comment

The Russian text is a simplified and shortened, retelling the original with omission of some sentences. A common feature of different kinds of plagiarism can be noticed here: some references (Chiari, Cruveilhier, Lang) were taken from the original, but the original itself is not cited. Referring to Eduard Lang, Lazovski changed the figure 29% to 20%. Moreover, "found in syphilitics" (Lang) is not the same as "of syphilogenic origin" (Lazovski).

Omission of some phrases and quotations caused alteration of the meaning: the opinion of Hans von Chiari (whose name is misspelled in Cyrillic letters making a correct phonetic reproduction impossible), given in the original within quotation marks, is represented by Lazovski as a fact. Meanwhile, the syphilis-related stomach ulcers continue to be discussed in literature [6-9].

Example 3

Werner Gerlach comments on the page 82 of volume 6, part 1 in Handbuch der Speziellen Pathologischen Anatomie und Histologie [2] about liver hyperemia (Figure 6.5):

> "Die alltägliche Form der aktiven Leberhyperämie, die den Klinikern seit langem bekannt, für den Physiologen eine Selbstverständlichkeit ist, dem Pathologen aber nicht zu Gesicht kommt, ist die Verdauung-shyperämie der Leber … kann sie pathologisch gesteigert und verlängert sein, ja zu einem Dauerzustand werden durch die Aufnahme von Spirituosen, durch reichliche Flüssigkeitsaufnahme, durch scharf gewürzte Speisen" [2].

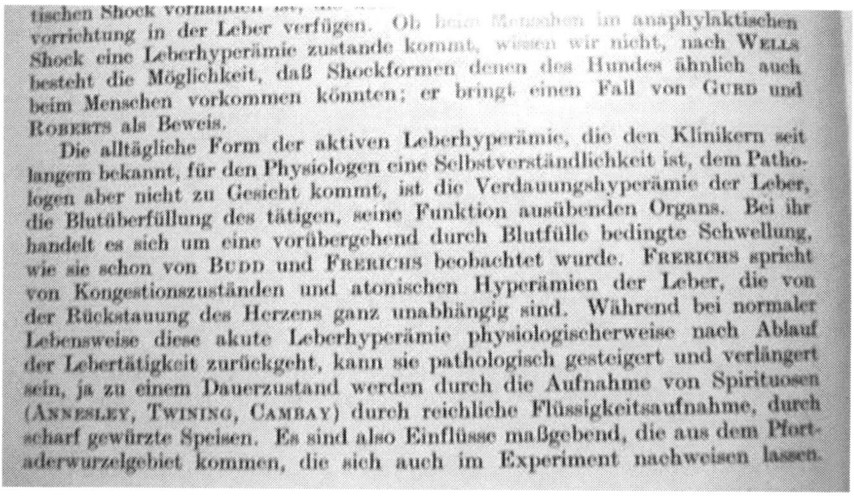

tischen Shock … vorrichtung in der Leber verfügen. Ob beim Menschen im anaphylaktischen Shock eine Leberhyperämie zustande kommt, wissen wir nicht, nach WELLS besteht die Möglichkeit, daß Shockformen denen des Hundes ähnlich auch beim Menschen vorkommen könnten; er bringt einen Fall von GURD und ROBERTS als Beweis.

Die alltägliche Form der aktiven Leberhyperämie, die den Klinikern seit langem bekannt, für den Physiologen eine Selbstverständlichkeit ist, dem Pathologen aber nicht zu Gesicht kommt, ist die Verdauungshyperämie der Leber, die Blutüberfüllung des tätigen, seine Funktion ausübenden Organs. Bei ihr handelt es sich um eine vorübergehend durch Blutfülle bedingte Schwellung, wie sie schon von BUDD und FRERICHS beobachtet wurde. FRERICHS spricht von Kongestionszuständen und atonischen Hyperämien der Leber, die von der Rückstauung des Herzens ganz unabhängig sind. Während bei normaler Lebensweise diese akute Leberhyperämie physiologischerweise nach Ablauf der Lebertätigkeit zurückgeht, kann sie pathologisch gesteigert und verlängert sein, ja zu einem Dauerzustand werden durch die Aufnahme von Spirituosen (ANNESLEY, TWINING, CAMBAY) durch reichliche Flüssigkeitsaufnahme, durch scharf gewürzte Speisen. Es sind also Einflüsse maßgebend, die aus dem Pfortaderwurzelgebiet kommen, die sich auch im Experiment nachweisen lassen.

Figure 6.5. Liver hyperemia. Reproduced from Handbuch der Speziellen Pathologischen Anatomie und Histologie,1930 [2].

This text can be translated as follows:

> "The usual form of active liver hyperemia, well known by clinicians and an obvious thing for a physiologist, but not encountered by a pathologist, is a digestive liver hyperemia... . It can be physiologically enhanced and prolonged, and even become a permanent condition,

because of alcohol consumption, abundant intake of fluids, and spicy food" [2].

The text by Abrikosov from page 228 of the handbook [5] is shown in Figure 6.6. It can be translated as follows:

> "Active liver hyperemia is not always reliably determined by autopsy. Clinicians and experimenters are however well acquainted with the rapidly developing and usually transient liver hyperemia. So, one can speak about digestive liver hyperemia that develops at a certain phase of digestion, especially after consumption of spicy food and alcohol…" [5].

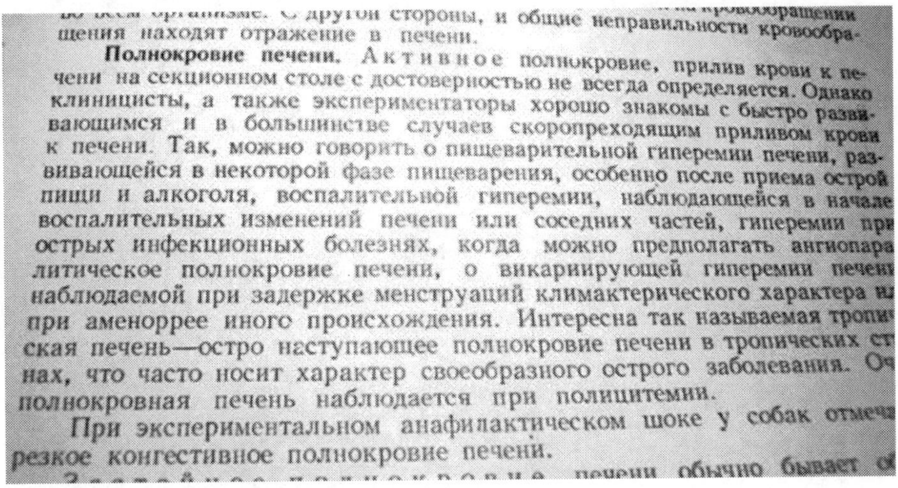

щения находят отражение в печени.

Полнокровие печени. Активное полнокровие, прилив крови к печени на секционном столе с достоверностью не всегда определяется. Однако клиницисты, а также экспериментаторы хорошо знакомы с быстро развивающимся и в большинстве случаев скоропреходящим приливом крови к печени. Так, можно говорить о пищеварительной гиперемии печени, развивающейся в некоторой фазе пищеварения, особенно после приема острой пищи и алкоголя, воспалительной гиперемии, наблюдающейся в начале воспалительных изменений печени или соседних частей, гиперемии пр острых инфекционных болезнях, когда можно предполагать ангиопаралитическое полнокровие печени, о викарирующей гиперемии печени наблюдаемой при задержке менструаций климактерического характера и при аменорее иного происхождения. Интересна так называемая тропи ская печень—остро наступающее полнокровие печени в тропических ст нах, что часто носит характер своеобразного острого заболевания. О полнокровная печень наблюдается при полицитемии.

При экспериментальном анафилактическом шоке у собак отмеча резкое конгестивное полнокровие печени.

Figure 6.6. Liver hyperemia. Reproduced from Mnogotomnoe rukovodstvo po patologicheskoi anatomii [Handbook of pathological anatomy in many volumes], 1957 [5].

Example 4

Gotthold Herxheimer comments on the page 938 and further on the page 944 of volume 6, part 1 of Handbuch der Speziellen Pathologischen Anatomie und Histologie [3] about cavernous hemangioma of the liver (Figure 6.7a,b):

sitzen, erkennt man sie schon an der Oberfläche der Leber, und zwar fallen sie hier durch ihre blaurote Farbe auf, ragen aber nicht über die Oberfläche hervor. Auf dem Durchschnitt erscheinen die Gebilde dann mehr dunkelrot. Sie sind im allgemeinen unter der Oberfläche von mehr halbkugeliger, im Organ von kugeliger Gestalt. Ihre Farbe weist schon auf ihren Blutgehalt hin, und in der Tat bleibt nach Ausspülung dieses ein weißes, schwammiges Gerüstwerk zurück. Nach außen sind diese Gebiete meist durch eine dünne bindegewebige Kapsel vom übrigen Lebergewebe abgetrennt, doch gibt es auch Kavernome, welche ohne eine solche in das Lebergewebe eingesetzt sind. Besonders bei den größeren ist jenes der Fall. VIRCHOW beschrieb schon diese Kavernome als eine „Substitution" eines gewissen Leberabschnittes.

Mikroskopisch bestehen die Kavernome aus Bluträumen, deren Wand zunächst (über die späteren Veränderungen s. u.) aus mit Endothel bekleideten dünnen bindegewebigen Scheidewänden besteht. In dem Bindegewebe finden sich hie und da auch glatte Muskelfasern, worauf schon VIRCHOW hinwies, und ferner elastische Fasern, zunächst in mäßiger Menge. Die Scheidewände hängen unmittelbar mit der das ganze Gebilde in wechselnder Dicke begrenzenden Bindegewebskapsel zusammen. Mitten in dem Kavernom finden sich häufig noch, wenn auch meist atrophische, zuweilen aber auch vikariierend hypertrophische (SCHMIEDEN) Leberzellbalken, wie dies vor allem SCHMIEDEN und RIBBERT betonen. Des weiteren finden sich in den bindegewebigen Scheidewänden hie und da Gallengänge.

Darauf daß diese Kavernome häufig in einer größeren Zahl in derselben Leber gefunden werden, will ich hier nur hinweisen; es ist unten noch darauf zurückzukommen. Ebenso darauf, daß sie sich auch schon bei Neugeborenen und kleinen Kindern finden, wenn sie hier auch meist kleiner sind und weniger ins Auge fallen. Daß sie bei Stauung der Leber infolge besonderer Blutfülle schärfer als sonst hervortreten, hat SCHMIEDEN betont.

a)

der Geburt. LUDWIG weist darauf hin, wie auffallend es ist, daß die Kavernome sehr häufig an der Konvexität des rechten Lappens in der Nähe des Ligamentum falciforme gefunden werden, d. h. in einer Gegend, welche gerade durch solche weitgehende Rückbildungsvorgänge ausgezeichnet ist.

Aus allen diesen neueren Behandlungen der Leberkavernome dürfen wir also wohl mit Sicherheit schließen, daß diese zunächst als Anlagefehler aufzufassen sind, aus fötaler oder postfötaler Zeit, und daß wir sie mit Recht als Hamartome oder Hamartien bezeichnen dürfen. Schließen sich echte Geschwülste an, so kann man auch von Hamartoblastomen sprechen. Wie steht es nun in dieser Hinsicht mit den Kavernomen? Diese Frage hängt eng mit der nach dem Wachstum der Kavernome zusammen. SCHMIEDEN beschrieb seiner Auffassung nach ganz beginnende Kavernome bei Neugeborenen bzw. wenige Wochen alten Kindern. Zunächst sind noch die Leberzellen erhalten; später kommt es durch Bindegewebswucherung zu der fibrösen Form der Kavernome. Er spricht ihnen jede besondere Neigung nach Art echter Geschwülste zu wachsen ab, lehnt daher für sie die Bezeichnung „Angiom" ab, hält vielmehr diejenige als „Cavernoma" oder „Naevus cavernosus hepatis" für richtig und stellt sie daher nicht in eine Linie mit den Angiomen der Haut und anderer Organe. RIBBERT andererseits, welcher ja die wenigstens sekundäre Ausschaltung aus dem Kapillargebiet der Umgebung stärker betont, hebt auch ihr weiteres Wachsen in das benachbarte Lebergewebe hervor, und zwar beschreibt er Sprossen, welche in dies eindringen. Allerdings ist das Wachstum in der Regel ein so langsames, daß Verdrängungserscheinungen an den umgebenden Leberzellen nicht zu beobachten sind. Dazu komme ein Wachstum per expansionem durch Erweiterung der Bluträume. Das Wachstum weise sich auch durch erhaltengebliebene Gallengänge in der Geschwulstkapsel aus. Ähnliche Wachstumsvorgänge an Kavernomen sind auch

b)

Figure 6.7a,b. Cavernous hemangioma of the liver. Reproduced from Handbuch der Speziellen Pathologischen Anatomie und Histologie, 1930 [3].

"Mikroskopisch bestehen die Kavernome aus Bluträumen, deren Wand zunächst (...) aus mit Endothel bekleideten dünnen bindegewebigen Scheidewänden besteht. In dem Bindegewebe finden sich hie und da auch glatte Muskelfasern, worauf schon Virchow hinwies, und ferner elastische Fasern, zunächst in mäßiger Menge."

"Aus allen diesen neueren Behandlungen der Leberkavernome dürfen wir also wohl mit Sicherheit schließen, daß diese zunächst als Anlagefehler aufzufassen sind, aus fötaler oder postfötaler Zeit, und daß wir sie mit Recht als Hamatrome oder Hamartien bezeichnen dürfen. Schließen sich echte Geschwülste an, so kann man auch von Hamartoblastomen sprechen" [3].

These two text fragments can be translated as follows:

"Microscopically, the cavernomas consist of spaces filled with blood with the walls formed primarily by thin fibrous septa covered by endothelium. In connective tissue can be seen here and there smooth muscle fibers, pointed out already by Virchow, and furthermore also elastic fibers, first time in a moderate quantity."

"From all that newer handling of liver cavernoma we can with certainty conclude that it should be primarily understood as a malformation from the fetal or post-fetal period, and that we can rightly designate it as a hamartoma or hamartia. Should a true neoplasm come in addition, it can be referred to as hamartoblastoma" [3].

The corresponding text fragments by Abrikosov from the pages 371 and 373 of the handbook [5] are shown in Figure 6.8a,b. The fragments can be translated as follows:

"Microscopically, the septa between the blood-filled spaces are formed of fibrous tissue with elastic fibers; sometimes with visible admixture of smooth muscle cells; the spaces are covered with endothelium" [5].

"Finally, some cavernomas result from malformation of hepatic tissue (Briukhanov), or from a separation, chorista, of vascular tissue, or hamaria in the sense of an excessive development of blood vessels in the hepatic tissue; in case of a considerable growth of such choristas and hamartias one can speak about choristomas and hamartomas ... . A possibility is not excluded that a vascular hamartoma acquires the properties of a true neoplasm, which is named hamartoblastoma" [5].

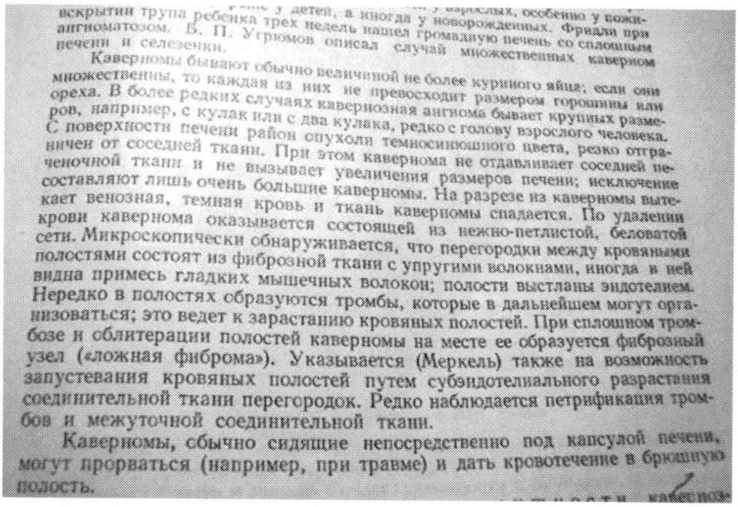

вскрытии трупа ребенка трех недель нашел громадную печень со сплошным ангиоматозом. В. П. Угрюмов описал случай множественных каверном печени и селезенки.

Каверномы бывают обычно величиной не более куриного яйца; если они множественны, то каждая из них не превосходит размером горошины или ореха. В более редких случаях кавернозная ангиома бывает крупных размеров, например, с кулак или с два кулака, редко с голову взрослого человека. С поверхности печени район опухоли темносинюшного цвета, резко отграничен от соседней ткани. При этом кавернома не отдавливает соседней печеночной ткани и не вызывает увеличения размеров печени; исключение составляют лишь очень большие каверномы. На разрезе из каверномы вытекает венозная, темная кровь и ткань каверномы спадается. По удалении крови кавернома оказывается состоящей из нежно-петлистой, беловатой сети. Микроскопически обнаруживается, что перегородки между кровяными полостями состоят из фиброзной ткани с упругими волокнами, иногда в ней видна примесь гладких мышечных волокон; полости выстланы эндотелием. Нередко в полостях образуются тромбы, которые в дальнейшем могут организоваться; это ведет к зарастанию кровяных полостей. При сплошном тромбозе и облитерации полостей каверномы на месте ее образуется фиброзный узел («ложная фиброма»). Указывается (Меркель) также на возможность запустевания кровяных полостей путем субэндотелиального разрастания соединительной ткани перегородок. Редко наблюдается петрификация тромбов и межуточной соединительной ткани.

Каверномы, обычно сидящие непосредственно под капсулой печени, могут прорваться (например, при травме) и дать кровотечение в брюшную полость.

a)

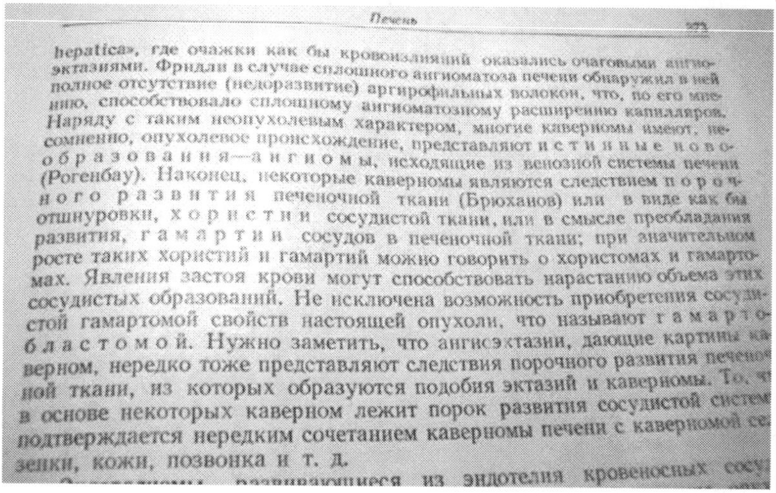

Печень

hepatica», где очажки как бы кровоизлияний оказались очаговыми ангиоэктазиями. Фридли в случае сплошного ангиоматоза печени обнаружил в ней полное отсутствие (недоразвитие) аргирофильных волокон, что, по его мнению, способствовало сплошному ангиоматозному расширению капилляров. Наряду с таким неопухолевым характером, многие каверномы имеют, несомненно, опухолевое происхождение, представляют истинные новообразования—ангиомы, исходящие из венозной системы печени (Рогенбау). Наконец, некоторые каверномы являются следствием порочного развития печеночной ткани (Брюханов) или в виде как бы отшнуровки, хористии сосудистой ткани, или в смысле преобладания развития, гамартии сосудов в печеночной ткани; при значительном росте таких хористий и гамартий можно говорить о хористомах и гамартомах. Явления застоя крови могут способствовать нарастанию объема этих сосудистых образований. Не исключена возможность приобретения сосудистой гамартомой свойств настоящей опухоли, что называют гамартобластомой. Нужно заметить, что ангиоэктазии, дающие картины каверном, нередко тоже представляют следствия порочного развития печеночной ткани, из которых образуются подобия эктазий и каверномы. То, что в основе некоторых каверном лежит порок развития сосудистой системы, подтверждается нередким сочетанием каверномы печени с каверномой селезенки, кожи, позвонка и т. д.

b)

Figure 6.8a,b. Cavernous hemangioma of the liver. Reproduced from Mnogotomnoe rukovodstvo po patologicheskoi anatomii [Handbook of pathological anatomy in many volumes], 1957 [5].

Comment

In general, the flow of ideas is identical to the original, while a deviation from it ("in case of considerable growth of such choristas and hamartias…") resulted in a questionable statement: the choristas (usually named ectopia or heterotopia) and hamartias, being developmental malformations, usually do not grow (or grow at the same rate as normal tissues e.g., in a child). A hamartoma is distinguished from a hamartia not on the basis of its growth but because of the tumor-like gross appearance of a hamartoma [10].

Example 5

The last example refers to the transliteration of the foreign authors' names in the Cyrillic alphabet with misspellings making difficult an even approximate phonetic reproduction. Figure 6.9 represents a quotation in the text written by Abrikosov, where the names of the foreign authors are given in Cyrillic letters without initials. The same in Latin letters would be: "Ribbert, Rössle, Gerlach, Hagerty, Devereux, A.I. Abrikosov" [5]. Note that some names (e.g., Devereux in Figure 6.9) are misspelled. Figure 6.10 shows the title page of this volume. Figure 6.11 shows the title page of Handbuch der Speziellen Pathologischen Anatomie und Histologie [1]. Abrikosov was a prominent Soviet functionary; and the librarians did not stamp or write on the title page of the book; all stamps and handwritten notices were made on the following page. This mechanism didn't work in case of the classical foreign edition, which is a bibliographical rarity in the former Soviet Union.

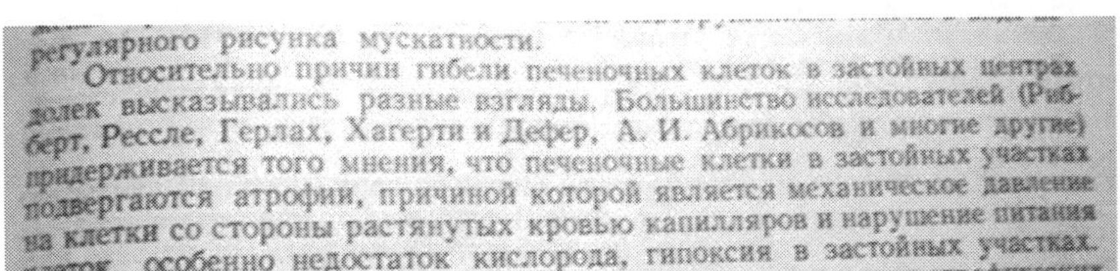

регулярного рисунка мускатности.
Относительно причин гибели печеночных клеток в застойных центрах долек высказывались разные взгляды. Большинство исследователей (Рибберт, Рессле, Герлах, Хагерти и Дефер, А. И. Абрикосов и многие другие) придерживается того мнения, что печеночные клетки в застойных участках подвергаются атрофии, причиной которой является механическое давление на клетки со стороны растянутых кровью капилляров и нарушение питания клеток, особенно недостаток кислорода, гипоксия в застойных участках.
Уже во второй стадии застойного полнокровия печени при атрофических

Figure 6.9. Example of quotation by Abrikosov: "Ribbert, Rössle, Gerlach, Hagerty, Devereux, A.I. Abrikosov." Some of the foreign names are misspelled in Cyrillic alphabet, making a correct pronunciation of the names impossible. Reproduced from Mnogotomnoe rukovodstvo po patologicheskoi anatomii [Handbook of pathological anatomy in many volumes], 1957 [5].

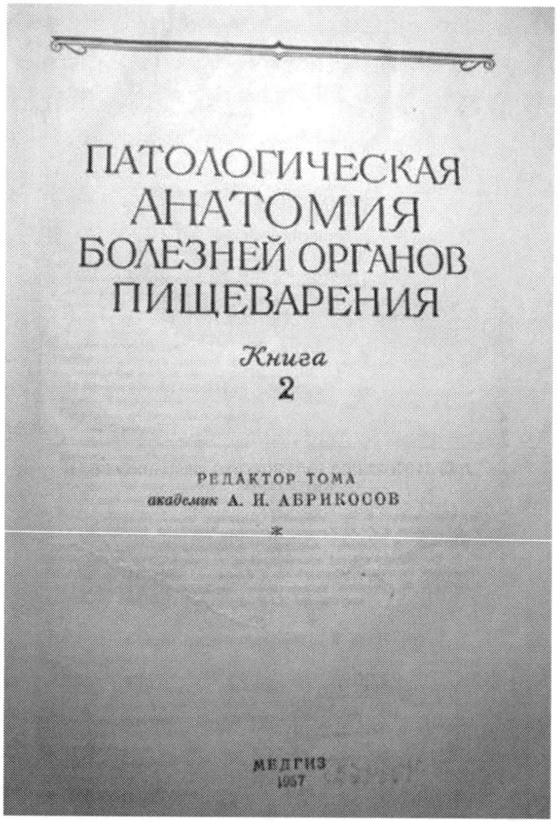

ПАТОЛОГИЧЕСКАЯ
АНАТОМИЯ
БОЛЕЗНЕЙ ОРГАНОВ
ПИЩЕВАРЕНИЯ

Книга
2

РЕДАКТОР ТОМА
академик А. И. АБРИКОСОВ

МЕДГИЗ
1957

Figure 6.10. The title page of the edition [5]. Librarians did not stamp or write on the title page of the book; all stamps and handwritten notices were made on the following page.

Thanks to the "Abrikosov's tumor", the name Abrikosov has become internationally known. In 1926 Alexei Abrikosov brought specimens from five cases for consultation to Otto Lubarsch (1860-1933), the head of the Institute of Pathology at Berlin University of Medicine (Charité). With the latter's support, there followed a publication in the Virchow's Archive [11]. The tumor was designated by Abrikosov as "myoblastomyoma" because of the similarity of its cells to myoblasts and topical relation to the striated muscle. In fact, the tumor had been described by Rudolf Virchow in 1854 [12]. The histologic images from the articles [11] and [12], morphologically similar, have been reproduced in [13]. The work by

Rudolf Virchow [12] was not mentioned by Abrikosov. Later on, histiocytic and nerve sheath cells have been discussed as probable progenitors of the granular cell tumor. Abrikosov was, together with Anatolii Strukov, an editor of the multi-volume manual for pathological anatomy (1957-1964), published by Medgiz in Moscow [4, 5], which largely followed the pattern of the Handbuch der Speziellen Pathologischen Anatomie und Histologie edited by Friedrich Henke and Otto Lubarsch, published by Julius Springer in Berlin (1924-1952); more details are in [14].

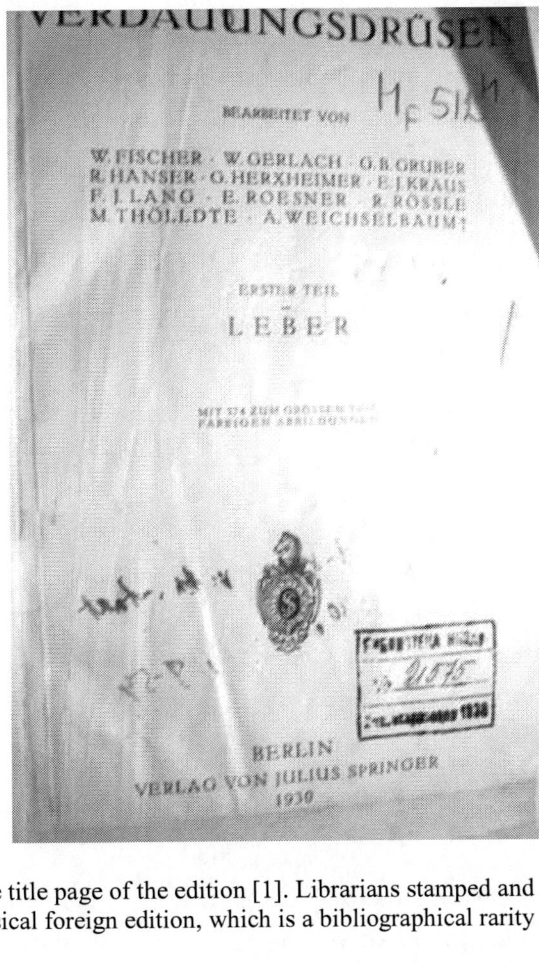
VERDAUUNGSDRÜSEN

BEARBEITET VON

W. FISCHER · W. GERLACH · G. B. GRUBER
R. HANSER · G. HERXHEIMER · E. J. KRAUS
F. J. LANG · E. ROESNER · R. RÖSSLE
M. THÖLLDTE · A. WEICHSELBAUM†

ERSTER TEIL

LEBER

BERLIN
VERLAG VON JULIUS SPRINGER
1930

Figure 6.11. The title page of the edition [1]. Librarians stamped and wrote on the title page of the classical foreign edition, which is a bibliographical rarity in the former Soviet Union.

Conclusion

The Pathological Institute of the Moscow I.M. Sechenov Medical Academy (recently renamed University) was situated until recently in a historic building in the Abrikosov Lane (Abrikosovski pereulok). It would be reasonable to rename it Henke-Lubarsch-Street, which would memorize the great work of these scientists presented to the whole humankind and to Russia in the first place, where pathology was studied predominantly after German sources at that time. It would also symbolize the new vision of a future international cooperation without plagiarism, misquoting, falsification, and other inappropriate acts in research and the publication process. Unfortunately, the Pathological Institute was relocated to a modern edifice in the 1990s, while in the old building major repairs and reconstruction were performed, the old interior was largely demolished and replaced by pseudo-traditional imitations [15].

References

[1] Konjetzny GE. Die Entzündungen des Magens. In: Henke F., Lubarsch O. (Herausgeber). *Handbuch der Speziellen Pathologischen Anatomie und Histologie.* Berlin: Julius Springer, 1928; Bd. 4, Teil 2, S. 768-1116.

[2] Gerlach W. Die Kreislaufstorungen der Leber. In: Henke F., Lubarsch O. (Herausgeber). *Handbuch der Speziellen Pathologischen Anatomie und Histologie.* Berlin: Springer Verlag, 1930; Bd. 6, Teil 1, S. 82.

[3] Herxheimer G. Lebergewächse. In: Henke F., Lubarsch O. (Herausgeber). *Handbuch der Speziellen Pathologischen Anatomie und Histologie.* Berlin: Springer Verlag, 1930; Bd. 6, Teil 1, S. 938, 944.

[4] Lazovski YuM. Zheludok [The Stomach]. In: Strukov AI. (Editor) Mnogotomnoe rukovodstvo po patologicheskoi anatomii [Handbook

of pathological anatomy in many volumes]. v. 4 *Patologicheskaya anatomia organov pishchevarenia* [*pathological anatomy of digestive organs*]. Editor of the volume A.I. Abrikosov. Moscow: Medgiz, 1957; book 1; pp. 281-551.

[5] Abrikossov AI. Pechen [The Liver]. In: Strukov AI. (Editor) *Mnogotomnoe rukovodstvo po patologicheskoi anatomii* [*Handbook of pathological anatomy in many volumes].* Moscow: Medgiz, 1957; v. 4, book 2, pp. 228-231; 371-373.

[6] Atten MJ, Attar BM, Teopengco E, Nadimpalli V. Gastric syphilis: a disease with multiple manifestations. *Am J Gastroenterol* 1994;89(12):2227-9.

[7] de Escalante Yangüela B, Lacasa Marzo J, Carrasquer Sese JA, Oncins Torres R, Palazón Astiz R, Sampedro Feliu JA. Gastric ulcers: a rare manifestation of secondary syphilis (in Spanish). *An Med Interna* 1993;10(6):287-9.

[8] Lichtenstein JE. Inflammatory conditions of the stomach and duodenum. *Radiol Clin North Am* 1993;31(6):1315-33.

[9] Rösch W. Ulcerative processes of the stomach (in German). *Leber Magen Darm* 1983;13(5):194-200.

[10] Müntefering H. Fehlbildungen [Malformations]. In: Riede U.-N., Wehner H. *Allgemeine und spezielle Pathologie*. Stuttgart; New York: Thieme, 1986; S. 256-78.

[11] Abrikosoff A. Über Myome ausgehend von der quergestreiften willkuerlichen Muskulatur [About myomata originating from the fasciated voluntary musculature]. *Virchows Archiv für Pathologische Anatomie und Physiologie und für Klinische Medizin* 1926;260:215-23.

[12] Virchow R. Ueber Makroglossie und pathologische Neubildung quergestreifter Muskelfasern [About macroglossia and pathological neoformation from fasciated muscle fibers]. *Archiv für pathologische Anatomie und Physiologie und für klinische Medizin* 1854;7:126-38.

[13] Jargin S. *Nachlass von Rudolf Virchow und die Stammzelle: ein Beitrag aus Russland* [*The heritage of Rudolf Virchow and the stem*

cell: a view from Russia]. GMS Medizin - Bibliothek - Information 2010;10:Doc14.

[14] Jargin SV. Historical examples. *Dermatopathology: Practical & Conceptual* 2010;16(3).

[15] Jargin SV. *Clinics of Moscow University.* Domus 7 Feb 2010 https://www.domusweb.it/en/news/2010/02/17/clinics-of-moscow-university.html.

Chapter 7

MANIPULATION WITH STATISTICS

INTRODUCTION

Below are presented several examples from the doctoral thesis [1] of the former Chancellor of Moscow I.M. Sechenov Medical Academy (1990-2009) Mikhail Paltsev, who was also head of the Department of Pathological Anatomy at the Academy. The academic degree "doctor of science" in Russia is supposed to be a counterpart of the higher doctorate in the countries, where this term is used, and to the habilitation in Austria and Germany. Numerous journal articles [2-14] and several books [e.g., 15] were published on the basis of this thesis. Summaries of many articles are translated into English and available on the PubMed.

Misinterpretation of statistical data and manipulation of statistics is a form of scientific misconduct, which was not uncommon in the former Soviet Union. By the end of the 1980s, some functionaries, predestined for high positions in scientific or educational hierarchy, published and defended as dissertations largely fabricated reports, containing provable falsifications and manipulation of statistics. A few specialists who had criticized such studies were dismissed from their positions.

Examples

The cover page of the dissertation by Mikhail Paltsev [1] is pictured in Figure 7.1. Figure 7.2 presents a table from this dissertation. In this table, the coefficients of linear correlation (r) are declared to be statistically significant and corresponding P-values are given. The level of significance (P) of a linear correlation coefficient (r) is defined by its own value and the number of correlation pairs (n). A comparison with the reference table [16] (Figure 7.6) has shown that almost all P values were invented. In Figure 7.2, the minimal values of the correlation coefficient (r), significant at the given number of pairs (n) according to the reference table [16], are handwritten in red. More details and translations are in [17].

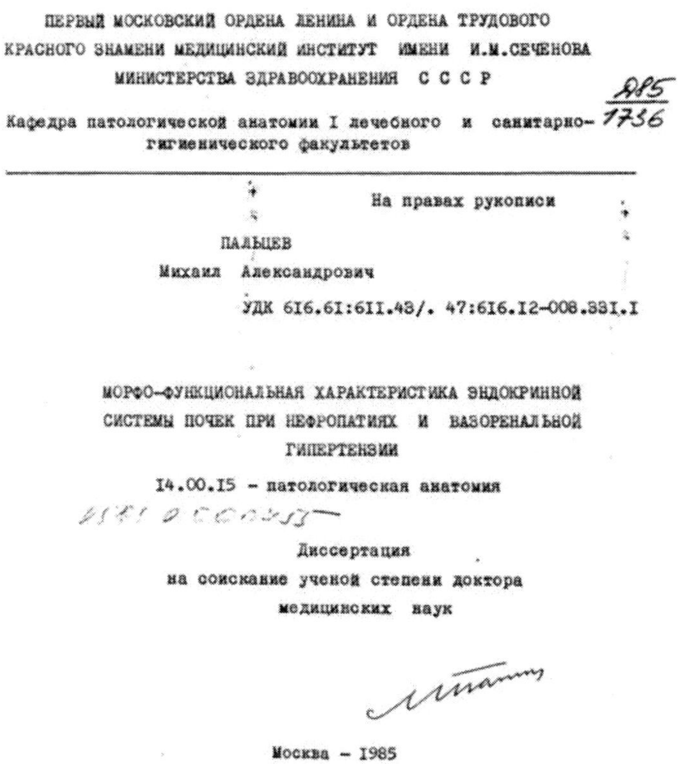

ПЕРВЫЙ МОСКОВСКИЙ ОРДЕНА ЛЕНИНА И ОРДЕНА ТРУДОВОГО
КРАСНОГО ЗНАМЕНИ МЕДИЦИНСКИЙ ИНСТИТУТ ИМЕНИ И.М.СЕЧЕНОВА
МИНИСТЕРСТВА ЗДРАВООХРАНЕНИЯ С С С Р

Кафедра патологической анатомии I лечебного и санитарно-гигиенического факультетов

На правах рукописи

ПАЛЬЦЕВ
Михаил Александрович

УДК 6I6.6I:6II.43/. 47:6I6.I2-008.33I.I

МОРФО-ФУНКЦИОНАЛЬНАЯ ХАРАКТЕРИСТИКА ЭНДОКРИННОЙ СИСТЕМЫ ПОЧЕК ПРИ НЕФРОПАТИЯХ И ВАЗОРЕНАЛЬНОЙ ГИПЕРТЕНЗИИ

I4.00.I5 – патологическая анатомия

Диссертация
на соискание ученой степени доктора
медицинских наук

Москва – I985

Figure 7.1. The title page of the doctoral thesis of the Rector of Moscow Medical Academy [1].

Таблица 26

Результаты корреляционного анализа морфометрических и функциональных показателей при хроническом пиелонефрите

№№ пп	Корреляционные пары	В целом: r ± m	P	n	Продолжительность течения хронического пиелонефрита, до 3 лет: r ± m	P	n	более 3 лет: r ± m	P	n
I.	F – S	0,35 (0,52) ± 0,09	<0,05	I2	–			–		
2.	F – БМ	–			0,36 (0,67) ± 0,I2	<0,05	9	–		
3.	F – ПБ	–			–			–0,44 ([illegible]) ± 0,05	<0,05	I
4.	F – Кр	–			–			0,54 ([illegible]) ± 0,06	<0,05	1
5.	F – Гр	–			– 0,43 ([illegible]) ± 0,I4	<0,05	8	–0,62 ([illegible]) ± 0,I0	<0,05	
6.	S – АДс	–			0,56 ([illegible]) ± 0,23	<0,05	I2	–		
7.	S – АДд	–			0,58 ± 0,22	<0,05	I2	–		

F – формпараметр; S – относительный объем интерстиция почки;
Гр – относительный объем гранул в цитоплазме эпителиоидных клеток ЮГА; АДс – систолическое и АДд – диастолическое артериальное давление; ПБ – продолжительность болезни; БМ – белок мочи; Кр – креатинин крови.

Figure 7.2. Table 26 from the dissertation [1]. Translation of the title: Results of the correlation analysis of morphometrical and functional indices in chronic pyelonephritis. Handwritten in red are the minimal values of a correlation coefficient (r), significant at the given number of pairs (n) according to the reference table [16].

Abbreviations [our comments are in square brackets]:

- r - linear correlation coefficient
- m - standard error of the linear correlation coefficient
- P - level of statistical significance of the linear correlation coefficient Translation of the explanatory notes under the table [our comments are in square brackets]
- F - form parameter [morphometric index, characterizing a degree of elongation or ellipticity of secretory granules in the juxtaglomerular cells]
- S - relative volume of renal interstitium [determined morphometrically in histologic specimens of renal cortex]
- Гр - relative volume of granules in the cytoplasm of JGA epithelioid cells [determined morphometrically on ultrastructural images]
- АДс - systolic blood pressure
- АДд - diastolic blood pressure
- ПБ - disease duration

БМ - urine protein

Кр - blood creatinine

Таблица 22

Результаты корреляционного анализа морфометрических и функциональных показателей при фибропластическом гломерулонефрите

№п/п	Корреляционные пары	n = 7	p< 0,05
1.	F – $АД_С$		0,65 ± 0,11
2.	F – $АД_Д$		0,51 ± 0,15
3.	F – S		–0,55 ± 0,35
4.	F – ЭПС		–0,60 ± 0,15
5.	F – Гр		–0,50 ± 0,19

0,754 minimal value of significant correlation coefficient

F – формпараметр; $АД_С$ – систолическое, а $АД_Д$ – диастолическое артериальное давление, S – относительный объем интерстиция, ЭПС – относительный объем эндоплазматической сети эпителиоидных клеток ЮГА, а Гр – секреторных гранул (ромбовидных протогранул и сферических гранул).

Figure 7.3. Table 22 from [1] titled Results of the correlation analysis of morphometrical and functional indices in “fibroplastic glomerulonephritis”. In this table, the coefficients of linear correlation (r) are declared to be statistically significant (P < 0.05) for all correlation pairs. The minimal value of statistically significant correlation coefficient for 7 correlation pairs (n = 7) for all pairs in this table) is r = 0.754 [16]; consequently, all P values are false and all correlation coefficients are statistically insignificant.

Abbreviations [our comments are in square brackets]:

F - form parameter

АДс - systolic blood pressure

АДд - diastolic blood pressure

ЭПС - relative volume of the endoplasmatic reticulum in the epitheloid cells of JGA

S - relative volume of renal interstitium

Гр - relative volume of granules in the cytoplasm of juxtaglomerular cells [determined morphometrically on ultrastructural images].

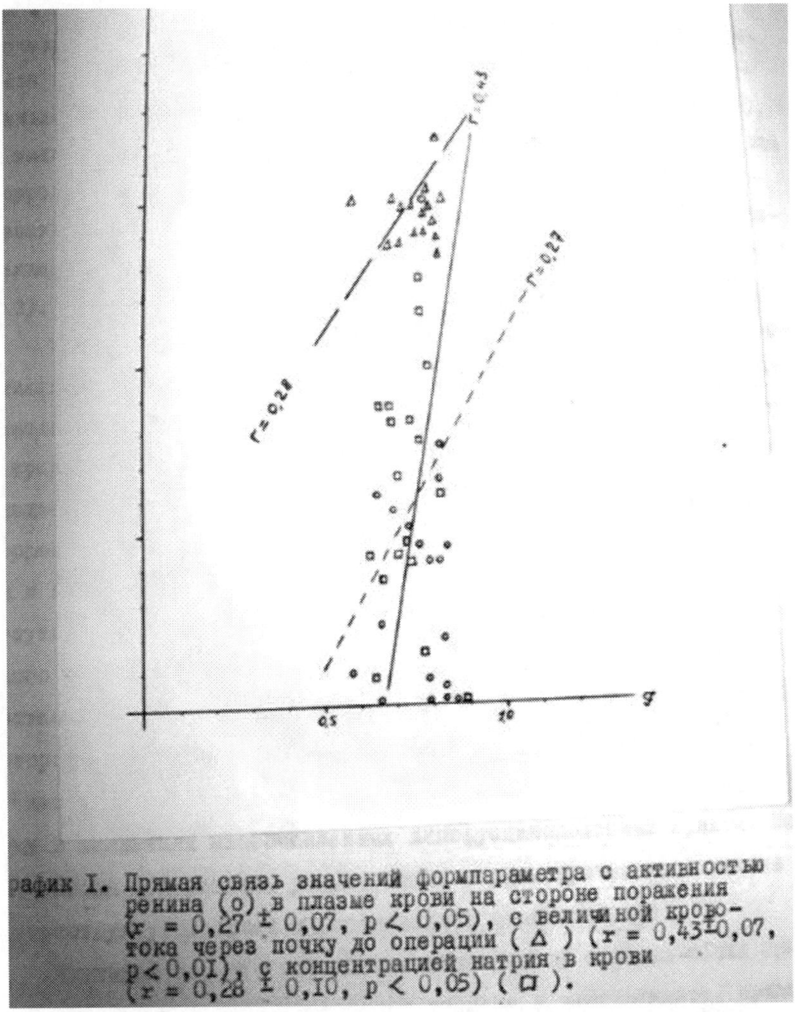

Figure 7.4. Graph 1, taken from the same source [1]. The translation of the explanatory note reads as follows [our comments are in square brackets]: "Direct correlation of the form parameter with renin activity on the stenosis site [in venous blood of patients with renovascular hypertension] (r = 0.27 ± 0.07, P < 0.05) (circles), with renal blood flow before the operation (r = 0.43 ± 0.07, P < 0.05) (triangles) and with sodium concentration in blood (r = 0.28 ± 0.10, P < 0.05) (squares)."

Comment: Three scatter diagrams together with all points are plotted on one graph. The calculation of statistical significance after counting the points has shown that all three correlation coefficients (r) are insignificant, and corresponding P-values are false. The numbers (n) of correlation pairs (or points on the graph): circles -19, squares - 18 and triangles - 16. The minimal value of a statistically significant coefficient of linear correlation for n = 19 and P = 0.05 is 0.46 [16].

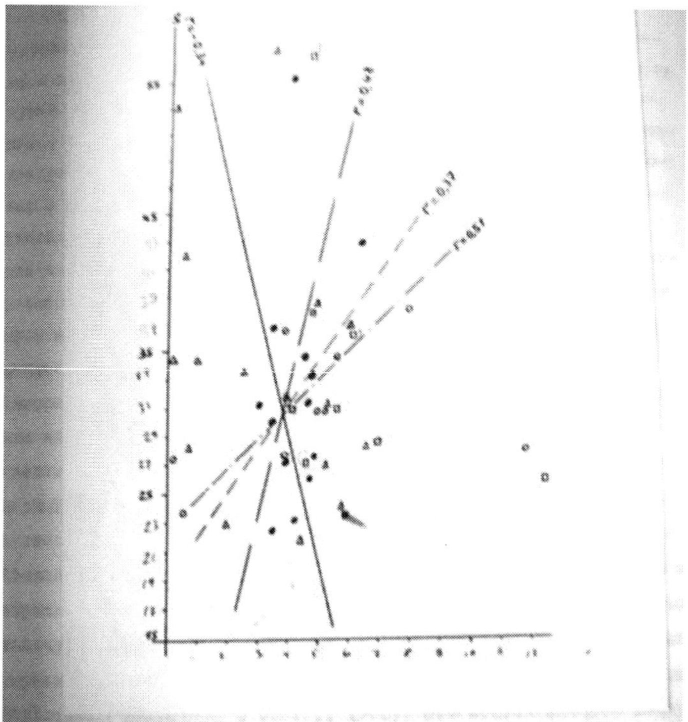

График 2. Прямая связь между площадью интерстиция и активностью ренина на стороне поражения ($r = 0,87 \pm 0,12$, $p < 0,05$) (○), а также величиной почечного кровотока до операции при продолжительности гипертензии свыше 3 лет ($r = 0,51 \pm 0,09$, $p < 0,02$) (□). Обратная связь между площадью интерстиция и величиной почечного кровотока ($r = -0,34 \pm 0,07$, $p < 0,01$) (△) и прямая связь с концентрацией натрия в крови ($0,48 \pm 0,09$, $p < 0,05$) (●).

Figure 7.5. Graph 2 from the same source [1]. The translation of the explanatory note follows below [our comments are in square brackets]: Direct correlation of the square of the interstitium [relative square of the renal cortical interstitium determined morphometrically on histological specimens] with renin activity on the stenosis site [in venous blood in renovascular hypertension] ($r = 0.87$, $P < 0.05$) (empty circles), with renal blood flow before the operation in cases with a disease duration ≥3 years ($r = 0.51$, $P < 0.02$) (squares). Inverse correlation of interstitium square with the renal blood flow ($r = -0.34$, $P < 0.01$) (triangles) and direct correlation with blood sodium concentration ($r = 0.48$, $P < 0.05$) (black circles).

Comment: Four scatter diagrams together with all points are plotted on one graph. The calculation of statistical significance after counting the points has shown that the three latter correlation coefficients (r) are insignificant, the given P-values being lower than they should be according to the reference table [16]. The numbers (n) of correlation pairs (or points on the graph): empty circles - 9, squares - 8, triangles - 15, black circles - 12. For example, the minimal value of a statistically significant coefficient of linear correlation for n = 15 and P = 0.01 (triangles) is 0.64 [16]. Note that all linear correlation plots, which are supposedly independent from each other, cross in one and the same point. It is extremely improbable and in itself is a proof of the data trimming.

Normalverteilung

Korrelationskoeffizient r: Signifikanz gegen 0*

2α ν	0,1	0,05	0,01	0,001	2α ν	0,1	0,05
1	0,9877	0,9969	0,9999	1,0000	101	0,1630	0,1937
2	9000	9500	9900	0,9990	102	1622	1927
3	8054	8783	9587	9911	103	1614	1918
4	7293	8114	9172	9741	104	1606	1909
5	0,6694	0,7545	0,8745	0,9509	105	0,1599	0,1900
6	6215	7067	8343	9249	106	1591	1891
7	5822	6664	7977	8983	107	1584	1882
8	5494	6319	7646	8721	108	1577	1874
9	5214	6021	7348	8471	109	1569	1865
10	0,4973	0,5760	0,7079	0,8233	110	0,1562	0,1857
11	4762	5529	6835	8010	111	1555	1848
12	4575	5324	6614	7800	112	1548	1840
13	4409	5139	6411	7604	113	1542	1832
14	4259	4973	6226	7419	114	1535	1824
15	0,4124	0,4821	0,6055	0,7247	115	0,1528	0,1816
16	4000	4683	5897	7084	116	1522	1809
17	3887	4555	5751	6932	117	1515	1801
18	3783	4438	5614	6788	118	1509	1793
19	3687	4329	5487	6652	119	1502	1786
20	0,3598	0,4227	0,5368	0,6524	120	0,1496	0,1779
21	3515	4132	5256	6402	121	1490	1771
22	3438	4044	5151	6287	122	1484	1764
23	3365	3961	5052	6177	123	1478	1757
24	3297	3882	4958	6073	124	1472	1750
25	0,3233	0,3809	0,4869	0,5974	125	0,1466	0,1743
26	3172	3739	4785	5880	126	1460	1736
27	3115	3673	4705	5790	127	1455	1730
28	3061	3610	4629	5703	128	1449	1723
29	3009	3550	4556	5620	129	1443	1716
30	0,2960	0,3494	0,4487	0,5541	130	0,1438	0,1710
31	2913	3440	4421	5465	131	1432	1703
32	2869	3388	4357	5392	132	1427	1697
33	2826	3338	4297	5322	133	1422	1690
34	2785	3291	4238	5255	134	1416	1684

Figure 7.6. A fragment from the reference table showing the significance of correlation coefficients against zero [16]. To find a minimal value of a statistically significant correlation coefficient, a column according to the P-value must be chosen, and a line - according to the value n-2 (n - number of correlation pairs). Using this table, we found out that some given P values are lower than they should be according to the reference table i.e., statistical significance was overstated in some papers e.g., [18].

Discussion

During the period 1982-1990 I was a trainee, thereafter pathologist and lecturer at the Department of Pathological Anatomy of the Moscow I.M. Sechenov Medical Academy, attended meetings of Moscow Society of Pathology, heard many scientific reports and defenses of theses. Along with reports having value of review or compilation, there were numerous useless and largely fabricated ones. Unreliable publications originated from renowned institutions. There was also some commerce around it: many postgraduates came to Moscow from other cities and Soviet Republics to be awarded a scientific degree; they paid for preparation of specimens, illustrations, and sometimes also for a review of literature. They also presented pricey gifts to their scientific consultants. Certainly, there was also serious research in some fields of medical science.

What are the implications of the unreliable or false data for the research and practice? It is difficult to evaluate the extent of damage, knowing only a limited amount of proven facts. Some risk for patients was caused by renal biopsies taken for scientific purposes in renovascular hypertension sometimes also from the contralateral kidney (opposite to the renal artery stenosis) [1, 4, 7, 8, 12]; more details are in Chapter 11. Invasive procedures applied without sufficient indications also for research are discussed in Chapter 10. As for the global science, there has been no appreciable harm: the studies discussed here have hardly ever been cited abroad. Their true scientific value has been understood by experts. The indirect harm has, however, been considerable: students and young researchers can learn from the Chancellor of Medical Academy that scientific misconduct brings success and profit.

Manipulations of statistics and plagiarism [19] have been proven in the present case; therefore, academic dispute would be hardly appropriate. Nonetheless, some speculations can be commented on: "Mathematical model of renovascular hypertension" [7, 8] "Renal endocrine system" and its "stereotype cyclic changes" in various renal diseases [9]. Corresponding English language summaries, available also in PubMed, deserve to be quoted in full:

"Comparison of the findings of clinical, instrumental, and laboratory examination of patients with vasorenal [i.e., renovascular] hypertension with the results of morphological analysis of renal bioptic material showed that multivariate regression analysis of the parameters of examination of the patients provides for authentic calculation of the quantitative index of nephroarteriolosclerosis - the vascular index of the afferent arterioles of the renal glomeruli. The calculated values of the vascular index for both kidneys are criteria for choosing the method of operative intervention in vasorenal hypertension." [8]

Comment: At that time I was employed at the same department and examined biopsy specimens from contralateral kidneys in renovascular hypertension; they were usually small, most of them contained no more than 1-3 glomeruli and arterioles, while many specimens contained none of these structures at all. Most of the specimens were unsuitable for a reliable morphometric assessment, let alone determining indications for the surgical treatment of renovascular hypertension. I informed thereof the chief researcher and other participants of the study, but they disregarded it. At that time I declined participation in a similar study, having said to the chief, the future Chancellor of the Academy, that I prefer to avoid partaking in falsifications.

Another summary [9] reads as follows:

"The renin-angiotensin (juxtaglomerular apparatus - JGA) and prostaglandin [interstitial cells (IC) of renal medulla and nephrocytes of collecting tubules (NCT)] systems of the kidneys were studied in 72 patients (renal biopsies, nephrectomy, morpho-functional correlations) with the nephrogenic arterial hypertension (vasorenal hypertension, chronic glomerulonephritis, pyelonephritis). Histologic and electron-microscopic methods were used; the renin activity was determined in the peripheral blood and blood from the renal veins. The results were analyzed mathematically and statistically using an original program. It is shown that stereotype cyclic changes develop in the endocrine renal system of patients with renal hypertension and that they reflect the stages of initial hyperfunction (ultrastructural hyperplasia of JGA cells with appearance of numerous immature granules; ultrastructural moderate hyperplasia of medulla IC; increase of blood renin activity), discoordination of functions (progressing JGA hyperfunction and depletion of prostaglandin synthetic function of medulla IC; compensatory activation of NCT; further increase of the blood renin activity) and depletion (atrophy and fibroblastic transformation of the JGA of the majority of nephrons and of medulla IC). The stages of renal endocrine system alterations in the arterial hypertension are the manifestation of compensatory and adaptive response. Morphofunctional analysis with the use of morphometry and mathematical statistics are necessary for the objective evaluation of this response." [9]

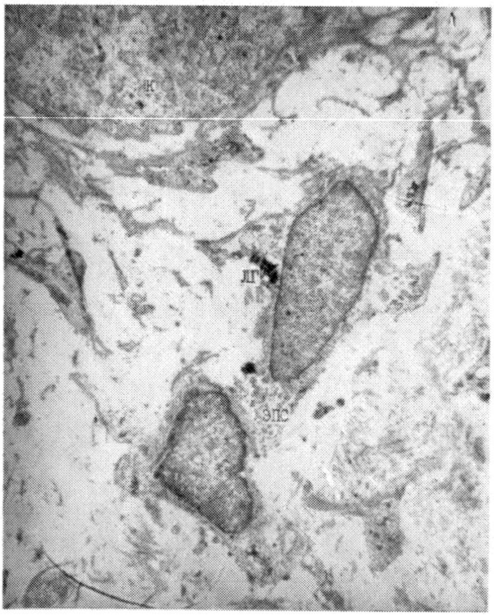

Рис. 78. Смешанная форма хронического пиелонефрита в период ремиссии без гипертензии. Умеренная гиперплазия эндоплазматической сети (ЭПС), липидные гранулы (ЛГ) в цитоплазме ИК в сохранных участках мозгового вещества. К – каналец. х 6 000.

Figure 7.7. Figure 78, an illustration from [1]. Translation of the explanatory note: "Mixed form of chronic pyelonephritis in remission, without hypertension. Moderate hyperplasia of endoplasmatic reticulum (marked ЭПС), lipid granules (marked ЛГ) in the cytoplasm of interstitial cells of preserved areas of renal medulla. Magnification: x 6000." It should be commented that structures marked ЛГ are probably artefects. Lipid granules in renomedullary interstitial cells have different ultrastructural appearance [20].

Comment: The quality of documentation of this concept is reflected by illustrations from the dissertation [1] (Figure 7.7 and Figure 7.8).

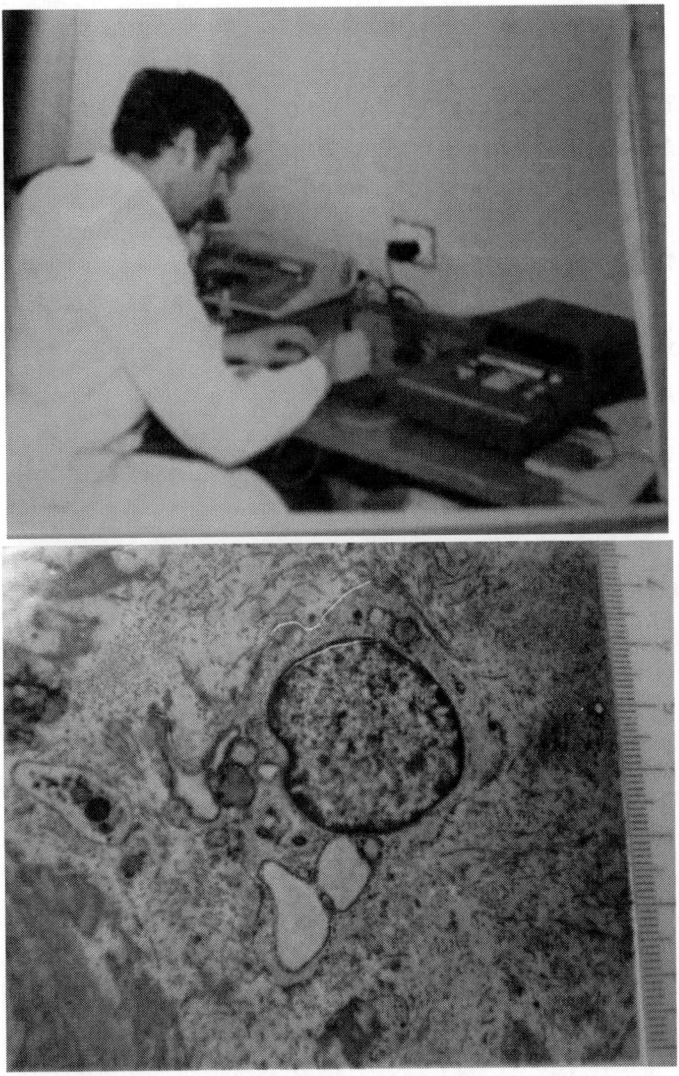

Figure 7.8a,b. a - Ultrastructural morphometry in action (year 1985). Left: Hewlett-Packard computer, right - image analyzing system; b - photograph of a renal interstitial cell used for ultrastructural morphometry. The cell membrane and some organelles are outlined by a ball pen connected to an image analyzing system. The cell membrane is not clearly visible.

In the late 1980s, I searched through the archive of ultrastuctural images on photographic paper and plates by Mikhail Paltsev and found approximately 20-30 images of juxtaglomerular cells with large quantities of secretory granules and rhomboid protogranules showing similar structure, probably originating from a limited number of patients and experimental animals. These photographs were used as illustrations in the dissertation, numerous articles and books. There was not enough material for a reliable statistical assessment of the "form parameter", relative volume of secretory granules, and other ultrastructural morphometric indices. Human renomedullary interstitial cells, bona fide suitable for assessment of prostaglandin synthesis, were absent in the Paltsev's collection. There were only a few doubtful ultrastructural images, similar to that in Figure 7.7, which were repeatedly used as illustrations in different publications. The phenomenon referred to in the above-cited summary as a "compensatory activation of nephrocytes of collecting tubules (NCT)" - a proposed morphologic equivalent of the enhanced synthesis of prostaglandins or other antihypertensive factors, has never been comprehensively illustrated. The data about "stereotype cyclic changes in the endocrine renal system" [9] in glomerulonephritis, pyelonephritis, and other renal diseases, and about the "calculated values of the vascular index for both kidneys as criteria for choosing the method of operative intervention in vasorenal hypertension" [8] have never been confirmed by other researchers.

According to [1], renal tissues from at least 96 patients with chronic pyelo- and glomerulonephritis underwent ultrastructural morphometry. Additionally, a large number of cases of renovascular hypertension (both kidneys) were reportedly analyzed. Corresponding quantities of representative sets of ultrastructural images never existed. I observed how this morphometry was performed: it was done by technical personnel using ultrastructural images on the photographic paper about 10 cm in size, by means of a ball-point pen connected to an image analyzing system (Figure 7.8a,b). Not much care was applied to this activity, which was sometimes performed during or after the alcohol consumption. Only the granule-containing cells were analyzed morphometrically; the mean level of granularity was not determined even for a single JGA, let alone representative assessment of different JGA from the same patient. Characteristically, secretory granules were measured together with nonspecific lipofuscin-like granules, known to be a "potential source of confusion when estimating the degree of granularity" [21]. Moreover, the common practice was selecting suitable images independently of their origin from one or another group, the single most important consideration being their fitting into the concept.

References

[1] Paltsev MA. *Morfo-funktsionalnaya kharakteristika endokrinnoy sistemy pochek pri nefropatiyakh i vasorenalnoy gipertenzii* (doctoral dissertation) [*Morphological and functional characteristic of the renal endocrine system in nephropathies and renovascular hypertension*]. Moscow: I.M. Sechenov Medical Academy, 1985.

[2] Serov VV, Pal'tsev MA, Kupriianova LA, Tankovich NI. The juxtaglomerular apparatus in chronic glomerulonephritis. *Arkh Patol* 1981;43(3):12-20.

[3] Serov VV, Pal'tsev MA. Endocrine system of the kidneys in nephrogenic arterial hypertension: functional and morphological analysis. *Arkh Patol* 1984;46(11):5-16.

[4] Pal'tsev MA, Serov VV. Endocrine system of the kidneys and nephrogenic hypertension. *Ter Arkh* 1987;59(8):110-3.

[5] Pal'tsev MA. Value of morphometry in the endocrine system of the kidneys. *Arkh Patol* 1987;49(1):62-7.

[6] Pal'tsev MA. Methodologic aspects of the interrelation between research methods in pathology. *Arkh Patol* 1986;48(12):3-6.

[7] Tankovich NI, Pal'tsev MA, Serov VV. Mathematical model of vasorenal hypertension. *Biull Eksp Biol Med* 1985;100(7):124-6.

[8] Pal'tsev MA, Krotovski GS, Egorova IA, Shcherbiuk AN. State of the neuroendocrine apparatus of the kidney during renovascular

hypertension as a criterion of the prognosis of the surgery outcome. *Arkh Patol* 1982;44(8):62-71.

[9] Pal'tsev MA, Bespalov DA, Shliapnikov VV, Kutyrina IM, Nikishova TA. Juxtaglomerular apparatus and interstitial cells of the kidney medulla in glomerulonephritis. *Arkh Patol* 1984;46(2):64-70.

[10] Serov VV, Pal'tsev MA. Neuroendocrine apparatus of the kidneys in disease. *Ter Arkh* 1982;54(7):14-18.

[11] Pal'tsev MA. Juxtaglomerular apparatus and interstitial cells of kidney medulla in hydronephrosis and chronic pyelonephritis. *Arkh Patol* 1982;44(5):12-19.

[12] Krotovski GS, Pal'tsev MA, Vinnitski LI, Turpitko SA, Shcherbiuk AN. Complex clinical and morphofunctional study of vasorenal hypertension. *Kardiologiia* 1981;21(7):62-66.

[13] Serov VV, Pal'tsev MA. Structural foundation for the functional connections of the endocrine apparatus and nervous system of the kidneys. *Arkh Patol* 1978;40(11):3-11.

[14] Pal'tsev MA, Bespalov DA, Shliapnikov VV, Kutyrina IM, Nikishova TA. Juxtaglomerular apparatus and interstitial cells of the kidney medulla in glomerulonephritis. *Arkh Patol* 1984;46(2):64-70.

[15] Petrov VI, Krotovski GS, Paltsev MA. *Vasorenalnaya hypertensia* [renovascular hypertension]. Moscow: Meditsina, 1984.

[16] *Wissenschaftliche Tabellen Geigy*. Basel: CIBA-GEIGY, 1980.

[17] Jargin SV. Manipulation with statistics in medical research. *Dermatopathology: Practical & Conceptual* 2009;15(1):21.

[18] Mukhin NA, Popova EN, Fomin VV, Popova IA, Kuznetsova AV, Ponomarev AB, Pal'tseva EM, Churganova LIu, Osipenko VI. [Clinical significance of markers of endothelial dysfunction and angiogenesis in progressing of the lung interstitial diseases] *Ross Fiziol Zh Im I M Sechenova* 2009;95(10):1139-50.

[19] Jargin SV. Examples of plagiarism from the former Soviet Union. *Dermatopathology: Practical & Conceptual* 2008;14(2):19.

[20] Venkatachalam MA, Kriz W. Anatomy. In: Heptinstall RH. *Pathology of the Kidney*. Boston: Little, Brown and Co., 1992. v. 1, p. 78.

[21] Biava CG, West M. Fine structure of normal human juxtaglomerular cells. II. Specific and nonspecific cytoplasmic granules. *Am J Pathol* 1966;49(5):955-79.

Chapter 8

FROM THE HISTORY OF RUSSIAN PATHOLGY

What has changed since the 1950s? The question can be answered using the example of the Department of Pathological Anatomy of Moscow Medical Academy, where I started as a trainee in 1982 and practiced until 1990. It should be commented that surgical and anatomic pathology is combined in Russia under the designation pathological anatomy. This department, which formerly belonged to the Medical Faculty of the Moscow University, has always been the leading department of pathology in our country. All main textbooks officially recommended for medical students and several handbooks have been edited by professors of this department.

Russian pathological anatomy originated and developed largely on the basis of classical German pathology. As discussed in Chapter 7, during the Soviet time some textbooks and manuals of pathology were partly rewritten from German sources. Such textbooks were re-edited with addition of own material repeatedly until 1993, when the last edition of the Textbook of Pathological Anatomy by A.I. Strukov and V.V. Serov appeared.

Professor Anatoli I. Strukov was head of the department from 1953 to 1972. In spite of his participation in the Stalinist reprisals against his colleagues and support of the notorious Lysenko-affaire, Strukov was known as a highly educated pathologist and good practical specialist. Under his guidance, much attention was given to the autopsy technique; trainees were taught to perform autopsies correctly and in detail. The histological laboratory was staffed with qualified technicians who routinely performed a dozen of histological stains and histochemical reactions.

Professor Victor V. Serov, an excellent lecturer and specialist in autopsy, a universally educated theorist, was head of the department from 1973 to 1990. During this period, a decline in the field of Soviet pathology became apparent. Autopsy was losing its academic profoundness. The head of the department gave up visiting the mortuary almost entirely. Obligatory postmortem investigation of all patients dying in the clinics caused an overload of pathologists specialized in autopsy (prosectors). The brain, bowels, and pelvic viscera were examined with decreasing frequency. Autopsy reports were written in a stereotypical pattern, while only the main lesions were described in accordance with the findings; microscopic descriptions of autopsy material were often invented. Postmortem diagnoses were sometimes adapted to preconceived ideas and formulated without sufficient evidence. Trainee pathologists were not regularly taught the autopsy technique, and were confined to basic methods.

The low salaries and social status of laboratory technicians have caused a shortage of these specialists. The quantity of available histological stains decreased; the majority of Moscow hospitals used the hematoxylin and eosin stain almost exclusively. The head of the department did not direct much attention to the biopsy diagnostics; this work was performed individually by several experienced specialists. Discussions of biopsy cases at the departmental conferences were seldom and rather formal; much more time was given to research and autopsy. Trainee pathologists were taught biopsy diagnostics only sporadically if at all. The technique of material reception (cutting up) remained primitive. For example, in cases of mastectomy or gastrectomy only 2-3 lymph nodes were usually embedded and sometimes no lymph nodes were found at all. There existed no written instructions for cutting up. Immunohistochemistry and other modern methods were available only for research and were not used on biopsy specimens even if directly indicated.

There was little development in the field of research. An impetus towards carelessness was given by the affairs of Lysenko and Lepeshinskaya https://en.wikipedia.org/wiki/Olga_Lepeshinskaya_(biologist), when authorities requested experimental evidence for false theories from scientists. Spurious ideas were imposed also in medicine (for example, the so-called theory of corticovisceral pathology and "ideas of Nervism") [1], the latter being confirmed by pathologists, who were encouraged to search for morphological substrata of various diseases in the central and peripheral nervous system. Since then the careless attitude towards reporting research results has persisted.

Candidate and doctoral theses as well as regular publications were needed to ensure a successful career. Limited technical possibilities and difficult access to foreign literature made the global novelty of research in the field of pathology hardly possible. At the same time, global novelty and practical significance were officially required from theses. This alone forced researchers towards biased presentation of facts and strained interpretations.

The most valuable studies in pathology followed this pattern: a large amount of foreign literature was studied and a meaningful concept was formulated. Original material was processed using modern methods, which were mastered. After the analysis of own results and the literature, conclusions were formulated and published, contributing to the dissemination of modern scientific knowledge and its adaptation to local conditions. It should be noted that even in such cases the principle of priority and even copyright was sometimes infringed upon because materials published by foreign authors were presented as original achievements.

In parallel, numerous useless and fabricated papers were published. Many scientists did not spend much time reading original articles and compiled their reference lists using abstract publications or reference lists from other articles. The misquoting was not unusual. The insufficient knowledge of the theory of statistics and lack of adequate controls resulted in the incorrect statistical assessment of data and manipulation of statistics in numerous scientific works. Plagiarism was widespread, while German sources were giving place to American ones. More details are in other chapters of this book.

By the end of the 1980s a new phenomenon became apparent: younger graduates, Party and Komsomol activists, predestined for high positions in the scientific or educational hierarchy, published and defended evidently fabricated dissertations, containing provable falsifications and manipulations of statistics; examples are in Chapters 1-7. Discussions of such reports at conferences transformed into public demonstrations of loyalty, because specialists understood the real value of such studies. A few experts dared to criticize these reports; some of them were later dismissed from their positions [2, 3].

Extensive changes of the Russian society in the 1990s affected also the field of pathology. The former Head of the Department, Professor Serov, always stressed the continuing academic traditions and the scientific school. Therefore, astonishing for many was the candidacy of his successor Mikhail Paltsev, the Head of the Communist Party Committee of the Academy. Paltsev had completed no postgraduate education in pathology and had never performed unaided autopsies or diagnostic investigations of biopsies. Decades have passed since then. The field of pathology in Russia has reached a more or less stable condition, which is acceptable for many. The leading pathologists have accumulated some knowledge as a result of their participation in lecturing and editing professional texts. The publication of dubious papers has continued; however, apart from their role in awarding scientific degrees, they have acquired another purpose: scientific institutions participate in the expert examination for the official registration of drugs and other medical products [4].

REFERENCES

[1] Strukov AI. Pavlovian physiologic theory in Soviet pathologic anatomy. *Arkh Patol* 1951;13(6):3-16.

[2] Jargin SV. Pathology in the former Soviet Union: scientific misconduct and related phenomena. *Dermatol Pract Concept* 2011;1(1):75-81.

[3] Jargin SV. Some Aspects of Medical Education in Russia. *Am J Med Stud* 2013;1(2):4-7.

[4] Jargin SV. Barriers to the importation of medical products to Russia: in search of solutions. *Healthcare in Low-resource Settings* 2013;1:e13.

Chapter 9

SCIENTIFIC MISCONDUCT IN PATHOLOGY

INTRODUCTION

In preceding chapters we presented several cases of plagiarism and manipulation with statistics in the former Soviet Union. Along with plagiarism, the partial isolation from the rest of the world gave rise to another phenomenon: extensive criticism of foreign publications. Here are presented several quotations from English summaries of Russian-language articles. The summaries are cited verbatim, exactly as they are printed in the journal.

> "Negative consequences of treatment are observed at least in 16% patients at multidisciplinary hospitals and may result from the causes that are independent of medical staff, but more frequently from errors and inadequate treatment standards due to human factors. Systematic improvement of professionalism, which should be started from some educational reforms at medical institutes, is needed" [1].

Comment: This is a review of foreign literature with extensive criticism of the complications of therapy and professional misconduct in medicine in the United States and other countries. Materials of the Agency for Healthcare Research and Quality, the National Patient Safety Agency, the American Iatrogenic Association, and other sources are used. Analogous phenomena in Russia are not discussed.

> "The experience by pathologists and clinical physicians in using the classification of tubulo-interstitial lesions of the kidney, which was developed in the 1980s, has shown that it adequately reflects the structure of this important section of renal pathology. At the same time the classification is proposed to be modified on the basis of the actual current spectrum of renal pathology." [2]

Comment: A critical review, written by one of the leading Russian experts in renal pathology, quotes only one foreign source, apart from two books translated into Russian. This reference is given without authors' or editors' names: "Renal disease. Classification and Atlas. Vol. 2: Tubulo-interstitial Disease. New York: Tokyo, 1982" [2].

Here follow several quotations (verbatim from Russian) from textbooks and manuals bearing official recommendations of the Ministry of Health. In the textbook of general pathology [3], officially recommended for medical students, extensive discussions against unnamed foreign authors are led:

> "Some authors declare that most important are local changes of organs and tissues, others advocate with the same persistence the paramount importance of general conditions of the organism… both do not see the main thing" (p. 26).
>
> "They [unnamed foreign authors] erroneously think that the final diagnosis was, is, and will be morphological" (p. 224).
>
> "…many large modern foreign manuals of general pathology provide little if any information about etiology, pathogenesis and theory of disease. They elucidate exclusively factual achievements of ultrastructural and molecular pathology, not trying to make broad generalizations." (p. 35) [3]

Another hallmark of this textbook is an extensive criticism of generally accepted terminology from the International Classification of Diseases, for example, such terms as ischemic heart disease, cerebrovascular disease (pp. 261-270), or some terms with the ending -itis, e.g., gastritis, pancreatitis, hepatitis (p.154), which is a hardly suitable discussion for a textbook for medical students. At the same time, neologisms are invented: functiogenesis, morphofunctiogenesis, amiloidoblast, amiloidoclast etc. [3] The next edition of this book [4] was enriched with plagiarism from Robbins' Pathologic Basis of Disease [5] (pp. 53-55 vs. 20, 27-29) and renamed Rukovodstvo (Manual) [4]. More details are in Chapter 2.

Former functionaries, promoted to high positions in science and education, do not always maintain a duly high level of educational publications. Some quotations from the Tests in Pathological Anatomy, an edition that was used at the Peoples' Friendship University of Russia, are presented below [6]. Outdated and erroneous information from this edition was noticed by students. We received no response to our letter to the Dean of the Medical Faculty (Figure 9.1). Verbatim translations from the tests:

> "Insufficient erythropoietic function of brain is a possible cause of anemia."
>
> "A focus of extramedullary hemopoiesis is named leukemic infiltration."
>
> "In exudative glomerulonephritis, serous, fibrinous or hemorrhagic exudate can accumulate within Bowman's capsule."
>
> "Chronic pyelonephritis is a disease with predominant involvement of glomeruli (glomerulopathy)."
>
> "Primarily contracted kidney is typical for arterial hypertension."
>
> "Reddish color of the liver in cirrhosis depends on the blood flow impediment in the portal vein."
>
> "Hepar lobatum belongs to infectious cirrhosis."
>
> "Abundance of mucus in the stomach is typical for atrophic gastritis."
>
> "Renal insufficiency (amyloidosis) is one of the main causes of death in chronic obstructive lung diseases" [6].

Translation of the letter (Figure 9.1):

Upper left corner: Registered 3.06.98; signature of the secretary at the Dean's office.

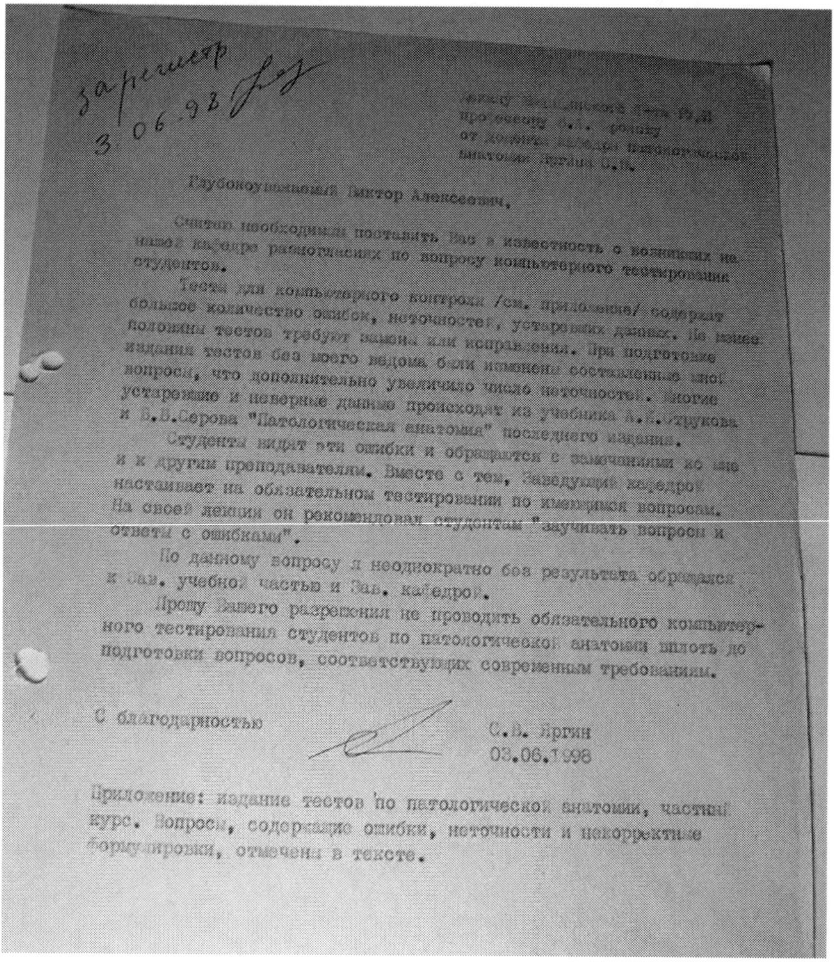

Зарегистр 3.06.98

Декану медицинского ф-та РУДН
профессору В.А. Фролову
от доцента кафедры патологической
анатомии Яргина С.В.

Глубокоуважаемый Виктор Алексеевич,

Считаю необходимым поставить Вас в известность о разногласиях на нашей кафедре по вопросу компьютерного тестирования студентов.

Тесты для компьютерного контроля /см. приложение/ содержат большое количество ошибок, неточностей, устаревших данных. Не менее половины тестов требуют замены или исправления. При подготовке издания тестов без моего ведома были изменены составленные мной вопросы, что дополнительно увеличило число неточностей. Многие устаревшие и неверные данные происходят из учебника А.И.Струкова и В.В.Серова "Патологическая анатомия" последнего издания.

Студенты видят эти ошибки и обращаются с замечаниями ко мне и к другим преподавателям. Вместе с тем, Заведующий кафедрой настаивает на обязательном тестировании по имеющимся вопросам. На своей лекции он рекомендовал студентам "заучивать вопросы и ответы с ошибками".

По данному вопросу я неоднократно без результата обращался к Зав. учебной частью и Зав. кафедрой.

Прошу Вашего разрешения не проводить обязательного компьютерного тестирования студентов по патологической анатомии вплоть до подготовки вопросов, соответствующих современным требованиям.

С благодарностью

С.В. Яргин
03.06.1998

Приложение: издание тестов по патологической анатомии, частный курс. Вопросы, содержащие ошибки, неточности и некорректные формулировки, отмечены в тексте.

Figure 9.1. Report to the Dean of the Medical Faculty of Peoples' Friendship University of Russia.

"To the Dean of the Medical Faculty of Peoples' Friendship University of Russia professor V.A. Frolov from the lecturer of the Department of Pathological Anatomy Jargin S.V.

Dear Victor Alekseevich, It was my duty to inform you about disagreement in our department in regard to the computer testing of students. The multiple-choice questions for computer testing (enclosed) contain outdated information, numerous errors and inexactitudes. At least a half of the questions should be replaced or corrected. In the process of

> preparation of this edition, some questions that I have compiled were changed without informing me, which additionally enhanced the number of inexactitudes. A great part of outdated or wrong information originates from the last edition of the textbook by A.I. Strukov and V.V. Serov "Pathological anatomy". The students notice the errors and make remarks to me and other lecturers. At the same time, the Head of the Department insists on the obligatory testing of students using these multiple-choice questions. During a lecture, he recommended to "learn the questions with the errors." This issue I repeatedly discussed with the Head of the Department and the Head of Studies.Herewith I ask for your permission to abolish the obligatory computer testing of students in pathological anatomy until the multiple choice questions will be prepared in accordance with the modern knowledge. With gratitude, Jargin S.V.03.06.1998
>
> Enclosure: Tests in pathological anatomy, special course. Questions, containing errors, inexactitudes and incorrect formulations, are highlighted in the text."

Previously we reported on scientific misconduct with the example of the Chancellor of Moscow I.M. Sechenov Medical Academy, Mikhail Paltsev, who simultaneously officiated as a Head of the Department of Pathology (named Pathological Anatomy in Russia) of the same Academy (Chpter 2). In 2009, Paltsev abandoned both his offices, but before doing so he provided employment for several functionaries (or their relatives), who had not much experience in research or practice of pathology. Some experienced specialists were dismissed to clear places for them, which was harmful to the quality of biopsy reporting and teaching. With time, the former functionaries accumulated some knowledge, and the system worked somehow. This phenomenon has been widespread since the late 1980s: many former Party and Komsomol functionaries were appointed into educational and scientific institutions. Among those employed by Paltsev at the Department of Pathology of Moscow I.M. Sechenov Medical Academy are the former Komsomol activist Andrei Ponomarev (a relative of Paltsev, according to some witness) and Yuri Kirillov, who had been a manager at the Ministry of Health responsible for pharmacological research. In the past, Kirillov used wedge renal biopsies, taken during kidney-preserving operations (e.g., lithotomy) from patients with acute or chronic pyelonephritis, for research of dubious quality; details and references are in Chapter 11. Some other lecturers and researchers of the Department were involved in scientific misconduct (E.A. Kogan, L.V. Lysenko, P.V. Yushkov, E.M. Paltseva and others). We wrote about these facts to the present Chancellor of Moscow I.M. Sechenov Medical Academy (recently renamed I.M. Sechenov First Moscow Medical University), Piotr Glybochko, but received no response. Extensive misquoting was demonstrated in the Glybochko's doctoral dissertation [7]; images and references are in Chapter 1.

Some publications, based on trimmed or fabricated data, are contradictory to the generally accepted knowledge and potentially misleading for the practice. For example, immunohistochemical evidence of the gene p53 mutation [8] was reported in all 36 studied cases of differentiated thyroid carcinoma, including 11 cases of follicular, 6 cases of papillary, 5 cases of medullary, and 14 cases of "papillary-follicular" (absent in modern classifications) carcinoma; whereas in all cases of adenoma and other benign thyroid conditions (26 cases) no evidence of p53 mutation was found (Figure 9.2) [9]. The resulting statistical significance of the difference is extremely high (36/36 vs. 0/26, $P < 0.0001$). In the literature, p53 mutation is regarded to be a relatively late event in the thyroid carcinogenesis, associated with undifferentiated or anaplastic carcinomas, usually not occurring in differentiated tumors [11, 12]. Therefore, the statement (verbatim translation): "High degree of expression of p53 in carcinomas and its absence in adenomas allows concluding that p53 can serve as a marker of thyroid carcinoma" [8] can be conductive to the overdiagnosis of malignancy, especially today, when the improved economy in Russia enables the purchase of modern immunohistochemical kits and to apply new laboratory methods. Our letter on this topic was rejected by the Arkhiv Patologii, which is the main journal intended for practical pathologists in Russia.

From M. Paltsev et al., Arch Pathol, 1998, No. 3, v. 60, p. 5-10

Expression of biomolecular markers in thyroid diseases Таблица 1

Экспрессия биомолекулярных опухолевых маркеров при заболеваниях щитовидной железы (ЩЖ)

Заболевание	Маркер							
	Ki-67		p53		c-myc		bcl-2	
	1	2	1	2	1	2	1	2
Рак ЩЖ (n = 36) carcinoma	36 из 36	14	36 из 36	45	36 из 36	5	36 из 36	6
Аденома ЩЖ (n = 12) adenoma	12 из 12	< 1	0 из 12	0	12 из 12	4	12 из 12	4
Аутоиммунный тиреоидит + рак (n = 9)	9 из 9	< 1	0 из 9	0	9 из 9	4	9 из 9	4
Окружающая рак ткань ЩЖ (n = 16)	16 из 16	< 1	16 из 16	< 1	16 из 16	5	16 из 16	4
Окружающая аденомы ткань ЩЖ (n = 5)	0 из 5	0	0 из 5	0	5 из 5	2	5 из 5	2

Примечание. 1 — число позитивных случаев, 2 — средний процент позитивных клеток (средний уровень экспрессии биомолекулярных маркеров). 1-positive cases; 2-mean percentage of positive cells

тоза. Здесь ткань железы имела тубулярное либо трабекулярное строение, капсула отсутствовала.

В 2 наблюдениях ФР ЩЖ и в 2 наблюдениях ФА ЩЖ окружающая опухоли ткань была неизмененной. В остальных наблюдениях ткань ЩЖ имела изменения, сходные с зобными: фолликулы были различной величины и формы, выстланы местами уплощенным, местами пролиферирующим эпителием. Ткань железы вблизи опухолево-

Экспрессия данного маркера в АИТ и аденомах была одинаковой, ниже, чем в карциномах, и составила 4 балла по общепринятой методике. Однако в окружающей аденомы ткани ЩЖ мы наблюдали самые низкие значения экспрессии — всего 2 балла (см. рис. 1, в).

Таким образом, высокие значения экспрессии c-myc в аденомах и в окружающей ткани могут

Figure 9.2. Table 1 from the article [9], commented in the text.

The access to foreign professional literature has been limited in Russia, which is harmful for the practice and research. The widely used manual of tumor pathology [13] is outdated, imprecise, and in many fields (bone marrow, lymph nodes, thyroid, soft tissue tumors, and others) is hardly suitable for diagnostics. Some passages from the section on thyroid tumors [14] deserve to be quoted:

In the section "Follicular Carcinoma" on p. 356, it reads: "In highly differentiated form [of the follicular thyroid carcinoma], cancerous elements more or less resemble the follicles of mature thyroid. They have different form and size; the covering cells can have hyperchromic nuclei, crawling onto one another like ground watch glasses" [14].

Comment: The term "ground watch glasses" (yadra v vide pritertykh chasovykh stekol), a mistranslation of "ground-glass nuclei," can be found in many Russian-language publications. It is a diagnostic criterion of the papillary thyroid carcinoma but not of follicular carcinoma. Nuclear changes, characteristic of papillary carcinoma, are not visible in the illustrations in [14]. In the section about follicular thyroid carcinoma, the most significant diagnostic criteria, such as the capsular and vascular invasions, are not mentioned; the images were reproduced in [15]. Using this most authoritative manual of tumor pathology, issued by the Cancer Research Center in Moscow, it is not always possible to differentiate follicular thyroid carcinoma from adenoma. This was one of the mechanisms of false-positivity of thyroid cancer e.g., after the Chernobyl accident; more details and references are in Chapter 12. For many pathologists, especially outside Moscow and Saint Petersburg, this two-volume edition [13] was for long time the main source of information on many topics. Another example from the same edition is found in the section on nasopharyngeal pathology [16], where no stromal atypia of nasal polyps [17] is described. We know of a case of a false-positive diagnosis of sarcoma as a consequence of this.

In the Atlas of Tumor Pathology [18] the following is written in the section about thyroid carcinoma (p. 402, verbatim translation): "In severe dysplasia appear cell groups with clearly visible atypia. Therefore, third grade dysplasia is considered as an obligate pre-cancer, which histologically is hardly distinguishable from carcinoma in situ. At the same time, it is believed that severe dysplasia differs from non-invasive cancer because it is reversible". Nuclear atypia (enlargement, hyperchromatism, pleomorphism) is not considered in the modern literature to be a criterion of malignancy in follicular and papillary thyroid nodules, and the concepts of dysplasia and carcinoma in situ are not applied to them [19]. Cases of false-positive diagnoses of thyroid carcinoma, caused by misinterpretation of nuclear pleomorphism as a criterion for malignancy, are known. The overdiagnoosis of thyroid cancer after the Chernobyl accident went along with the overtreatment i.e., excessively radical surgery and radiotherapy; details and references are in Chapter 12.

Thanks to the economic upturn in Russia, some institutions started purchasing foreign literature. On the other hand, the acquisition of literature by medical libraries has decreased since the 1980s [20]. Many articles have become available online these days. Nonetheless, foreign publications are scarcely quoted in certain Russian-language articles; well-known phenomena, disease entities, morphological changes etc. are described without referring to foreign publications, which can be misunderstood as a global novelty [21, 22]. Here follow two quotations from English summaries of articles published in the journal Arkhiv Patologii. The summaries are available on the PubMed.

> "The structure, clinical manifestations, behavior of cavernous hemangioma of the skin of the face and neck, and the oral soft tissues were studied, by using biopsy specimens from 229 patients. Three types of cavernous hemangioma of these areas were identified. Their preferred treatments were defined and pathogenetically warranted" [23].

Comment: describing such a well-known lesion as cutaneous hemangioma, the authors did not quote a single foreign source. The 3-volume Pathological Anatomy by Paltsev and Anichkov [24], largely re-written from Robbins' Pathologic Basis of Disease, is quoted instead; details and evidence are in Chapter 2.

Another example reads: "The authors present the incidence and specific features of specific bone marrow lesion and the state of normal hemopoiesis and stroma. The criteria for the differential diagnosis of reactive polyclonal lymphoid proliferation in the bone marrow that may accompany many haematological and non-haematological diseases with specific bone marrow lesion in lymphoproliferative diseases are outlined" and further: "According to our results, several histological types of bone marrow involvement in lymphoproliferative diseases can be distinguished: diffuse, interstitial and focal" [25]. Then follows the usual description of the bone marrow involvement patterns by lymphoma that can be found in many textbooks, which are not referenced. The text can be misunderstood as an original description of bone marrow involvement patterns by lymphoproliferative disorders.

DISCUSSION

Scientific misconduct in the Soviet science has its history. The 1949 Session of Agricultural Academy of the USSR was a significant event for biology and medicine. Two false theories were forced through at this Session and during following years. First, is Trofim Lysenko's theory about inheritance of environmentally acquired features (https://en.wikipedia.org/wiki/Trofim_Lysenko), while genetics was labeled as a pseudo-science. Second, the “discovery” by Olga Lepeshinskaia about de novo formation of living cells in amorphous substances without precursor cells e.g., in the egg-yolk or detritus from wounds. Obviously, experimental evidence in support of these theories could be obtained only by means of fabrication. Besides, the so-called Nervism ideas (a derivative of Ivan Pavlov’s teaching about central role of the nervous system) were propagated. Pathologists were encouraged to search for morphological substrates of different diseases in the central and peripheral nervous system. Accordingly, such substrates were found and described, while pathogenetic significance of unspecific or accidental changes was often overvalued. Corresponding data persisted in the textbooks till the mid-1990s.

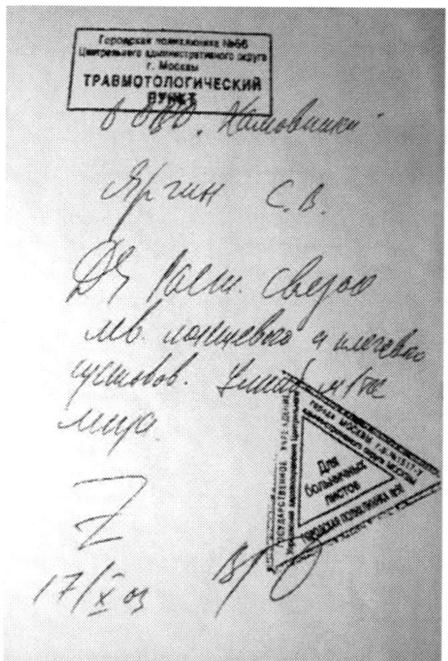
г. Москвы
ТРАВМОТОЛОГИЧЕСКИЙ
Яргин С.В.
17/X 03

Figure 9.3. Certificate from the trauma station. Translation: Rectangular stamp: City Polyclinic No. 56 of the Central Administrative District, city of Moscow. Trauma Station. To the Department of Home Affairs “Khamovniki” Jargin S.V. Diagnosis: sprain of the ligaments of the left elbow and shoulder joints; injury of soft tissues of the face. 17.10.2003. Signature. Triangular stamp of the City Polyclinic No. 56.

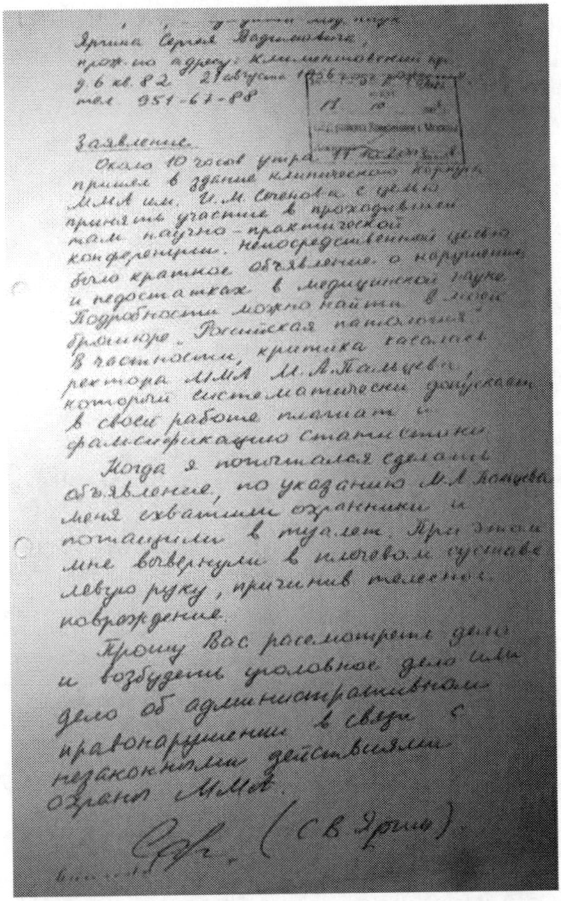

Ярина Сергея Вадимовича,
прож. по адресу: Климентовский пер.
д. 6 кв. 82 21 августа 1956 года рождения
тел. 951-67-88

Заявление

Около 10 часов утра 17.10.2003 я пришел в здание клинического корпуса ММА им. И.М. Сеченова с целью принять участие в проходившей там научно-практической конференции. Непосредственной целью было краткое объявление о нарушениях и недостатках в медицинской науке. Подробности можно найти в моей брошюре „Российская патология". В частности, критика касалась ректора ММА М.А. Пальцева, который систематически допускает в своей работе плагиат и фальсификацию статистики.

Когда я попытался сделать объявление, по указанию М.А. Пальцева меня схватили охранники и потащили в туалет. При этом мне вывернули в плечевом суставе левую руку, причинив телесное повреждение.

Прошу Вас рассмотреть дело и возбудить уголовное дело или дело об административном правонарушении в связи с незаконными действиями охраны ММА.

(С.В. Ярин)

Figure 9.4. The report to the Police (militia). Translation: Rectangular stamp: registered No. Illegible 17.10.2003. From the candidate of medical sciences Jargin Sergei Vadimovich, residing at the address: Clementovski per, house 6, apartment 82; born on 21.08.1956; telephone: 9516788 Report On 17.10.2003 around 10 a.m. I came to the clinical building of the I.M. Sechenov Moscow Medical Academy (MMA) in order to participate at the scientific and practical conference that took place there. My immediate purpose was making a short announcement about inappropriate acts in medical science. Details can be found in my booklet "Russian Pathology." In particular, the criticism was directed against the Chancellor of the MMA Mikhail Paltsev, who applies plagiarism and falsification of statistics in his work. When I tried to make the announcement, by instruction of Paltsev, security guards seized me and dragged to the toilet. In doing this, they twisted my left arm, having inflicted an injury. Herewith I ask to examine the case and to institute criminal proceedings or an investigation of a civil tort because of unlawful acts committed by security guards of the MMA. Signature.

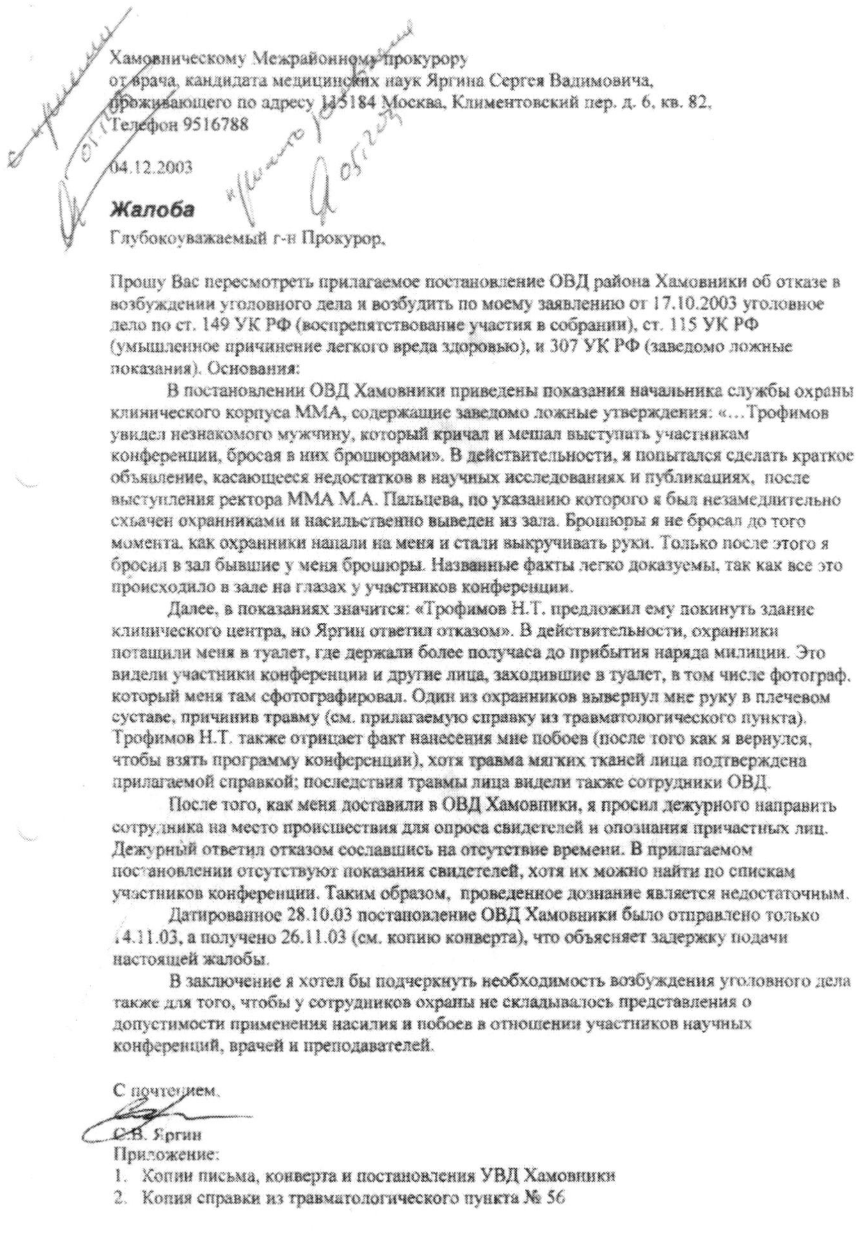

Хамовническому Межрайонному прокурору
от врача, кандидата медицинских наук Яргина Сергея Вадимовича,
проживающего по адресу 115184 Москва, Климентовский пер. д. 6, кв. 82,
Телефон 9516788

04.12.2003

Жалоба

Глубокоуважаемый г-н Прокурор,

Прошу Вас пересмотреть прилагаемое постановление ОВД района Хамовники об отказе в возбуждении уголовного дела и возбудить по моему заявлению от 17.10.2003 уголовное дело по ст. 149 УК РФ (воспрепятствование участия в собрании), ст. 115 УК РФ (умышленное причинение легкого вреда здоровью), и 307 УК РФ (заведомо ложные показания). Основания:

В постановлении ОВД Хамовники приведены показания начальника службы охраны клинического корпуса ММА, содержащие заведомо ложные утверждения: «…Трофимов увидел незнакомого мужчину, который кричал и мешал выступать участникам конференции, бросая в них брошюрами». В действительности, я попытался сделать краткое объявление, касающееся недостатков в научных исследованиях и публикациях, после выступления ректора ММА М.А. Пальцева, по указанию которого я был незамедлительно схвачен охранниками и насильственно выведен из зала. Брошюры я не бросал до того момента, как охранники напали на меня и стали выкручивать руки. Только после этого я бросил в зал бывшие у меня брошюры. Названные факты легко доказуемы, так как все это происходило в зале на глазах у участников конференции.

Далее, в показаниях значится: «Трофимов Н.Т. предложил ему покинуть здание клинического центра, но Яргин ответил отказом». В действительности, охранники потащили меня в туалет, где держали более получаса до прибытия наряда милиции. Это видели участники конференции и другие лица, заходившие в туалет, в том числе фотограф, который меня там сфотографировал. Один из охранников вывернул мне руку в плечевом суставе, причинив травму (см. прилагаемую справку из травматологического пункта). Трофимов Н.Т. также отрицает факт нанесения мне побоев (после того как я вернулся, чтобы взять программу конференции), хотя травма мягких тканей лица подтверждена прилагаемой справкой; последствия травмы лица видели также сотрудники ОВД.

После того, как меня доставили в ОВД Хамовники, я просил дежурного направить сотрудника на место происшествия для опроса свидетелей и опознания причастных лиц. Дежурный ответил отказом сославшись на отсутствие времени. В прилагаемом постановлении отсутствуют показания свидетелей, хотя их можно найти по спискам участников конференции. Таким образом, проведенное дознание является недостаточным.

Датированное 28.10.03 постановление ОВД Хамовники было отправлено только 14.11.03, а получено 26.11.03 (см. копию конверта), что объясняет задержку подачи настоящей жалобы.

В заключение я хотел бы подчеркнуть необходимость возбуждения уголовного дела также для того, чтобы у сотрудников охраны не складывалось представления о допустимости применения насилия и побоев в отношении участников научных конференций, врачей и преподавателей.

С почтением,

С.В. Яргин

Приложение:

1. Копии письма, конверта и постановления УВД Хамовники
2. Копия справки из травматологического пункта № 56

Figure 9.5. The report to the prosecution office. Translation of the last paragraph: "In conclusion I would like to stress that criminal proceding is important in this case because security guards should not think that they may apply violence, assault and battery to participants of scientific conferences, doctors and lecturers."

Our articles with criticism of scientific misconduct were rejected by the journal Arkhiv Patologii (Archives of Pathology). The attempts to make presentations at conferences were met with obstruction and violence; for example, on October 17, 2003 at the conference "Diagnostic Radiology and Scientific-Technical Progress" on the premises of Moscow I.M. Sechenov Medical Academy. The Chairmen at the Conference were Mikhail Paltsev, the chancellor of I.M. Sechenov Medical Academy, and Yevgeniy Chazov (https://en.wikipedia.org/wiki/Yevgeniy_Chazov), director of the Cardiology Research Center in Moscow and the former health minister. Dubious publications by Chazov and co-workers [26] were commented last in [27]. I tried to make a short announcement at the Conference, but was forcibly removed by security personnel, while mild injuries were inflicted, confirmed by a certificate from a trauma station of a Polyclinic (Figure 9.3). The case was reported to the authorities (Figures 9-4, 5).

CONCLUSION

There is a persisting interest in the topic of scientific misconduct. The following main forms of scientific misconduct are known: plagiarism, falsification or fabrication of data, manipulations with statistics, misquoting, false or gift authorship, as well as revenge on the whistleblowers revealing and exposing such cases. Former functionaries, their relatives and protegees, promoted to high positions in academies and universities in the former Soviet Union, are often unable to maintain duly high academic standards. Some textbooks, manuals and journal articles are imprecise, contain plagiarism or misleading information that may be conductive e.g., to the overdiagnosis of malignancy. However, in spite of shortages and drawbacks, there are grounds for optimism. The upturn of the economy in Russia makes possible the purchase of foreign literature and modern equipment, introducing new methods into research and practice. Therefore, we hope that this chapter will be only of historical interest in the near future.

References

[1] Vovk EI, Vertkin AL, Zairatyants OV, Frolova YuV. Foreign experience in registering and analyzing the poor outcomes of treatment. *Arkh Patol* 2007;69(5):16-24.

[2] Perov YL. Tubular interstitial pathology of the kidney (on the 25th anniversary of the WHO Expert Committee Classification). *Arkh Patol* 2008;70(1):13-16.

[3] Sarkisov DS, Paltsev MA, Khitrov NK. *Obshaya patologiya cheloveka* [*Human general pathology*] Moscow: Meditsina, 1995.

[4] Paltsev MA, Khitrov NK. Patologiya kletki. Distrofiya, atrofiya i nekroz [Dystrophy, atrophy and necrosis] In: Khitrov NK, Sarkisov DS, Paltsev MA, editors. *Rukovodstvo po obshey patologii cheloveka* [*Manual of human general pathology*] Moscow: Meditsina, 1999. pp. 42-67.

[5] Cotran RS, Kumar V, Robbins SL. *Robbins' Pathologic Basis of Disease.* Philadelphia: W.B. Saunders Co., 1989.

[6] Babichenko II, Vladimirtseva AL, Gundorova LV, Kharchenko NM, Jargin SV. *Testy po patologicheskoy anatomii. Chastniy kurs* [*Tests in pathological anatomy. Special course*] Moscow: Peoples' Friensdhip University of Russia, 1997. Available at: https://www.researchgate.net/publication/280829116_Testy_po_patologiceskoj_anatomii_Castnyj_kurs

[7] Glybochko PV. *Treatment optimization of benign prostatic hyperplasia combined with senile osteoporosis.* Doctoral dissertation. Saratov, 2001. (in Russian)

[8] Paltsev MA, Kogan EA, Tuntsova OI. Immunohistochemistry of biomolecular markers of early thyroid cancer. *Arkh Patol* 1997;59(6):18-23.

[9] Paltsev MA, Kogan EA, Tuntsova OI, Severin ES, Silaeva SA, Golenchenko VA. Morphological and molecular-genetic characteristics of carcinoma, adenoma and surrounding tissue of the thyroid gland. *Arkh Patol* 1998;60(3):5-10.

[10] Paltsev MA, Kogan EA, Tuntsova OV. Molecular markers of early thyroid cancer. *Path Res Pract* 1997;193:390. (abstract P191)

[11] Soares P, Sobrinho-Simões M. Recent advances in cytometry, cytogenetics and molecular genetics in thyroid tumors and tumor-like lesions. *Path Res Pract* 1995;191:304-17.

[12] Suáres HG. Genetic alterations in human epithelial thyroid tumours. *Clin Endocrinol* 1998;48:531-6.

[13] Krayevskiy NA, Smolyannikov AV, Sarkisov DS, editors. *Patologo-anatomicheskaya diagnostika opucholey cheloveka [Pathologo-anatomic diagnostics of human tumors].* Moskow: Meditsina, 1993.

[14] Goldburt NN. Opukholi shchitovidnoi zhelezy [Thyroid tumors] In: Krayevskiy NA, Smolyannikov AV, Sarkisov DS, editors. *Patologo-anatomicheskaya diagnostika opucholey cheloveka [Pathologo-anatomic diagnostics of human tumors*]. Vol. 2. Moskow: Meditsina, 1993. pp. 349-62.

[15] Jargin SV. Pathology in the former Soviet Union: scientific misconduct and related phenomena. *Dermatol Pract Concept* 2011;1(1):75-81.

[16] Bykova VP. Opukholi polosti nosa, okolonosovykh pazukh i nosoglotki [Tumors of nasal cavity, paranasal sinuses, and nasopharynx] In: Krayevskiy NA, Smolyannikov AV, Sarkisov DS, editors. *Patologo-anatomicheskaya diagnostika opucholey cheloveka* [*Pathologo-anatomic diagnostics of human tumors*] Vol. 1. Moskow: Meditsina, 1993. pp. 409-36.

[17] Mills SE, Fechner RE. The nose, paranasal sinuses, and nasopharynx. In: Sternberg SS, editor. *Diagnostic Surgical Pathology*. Vol. 2. New York: Raven Press, 1989. pp. 663-4.

[18] Paltsev MA, Anichkov NM. *Atlas patologii opukholei cheloveka* [*Atlas of human tumor pathology*] Moscow: Meditsina; 2005. p. 402.

[19] Rosai J. *Rosai and Ackerman's Surgical Pathology*. Vol. 1. Edinburgh: Mosby, 2004. pp. 515-94.

[20] Jargin SV. The state of medical libraries in the former Soviet Union. *Health Info Libr J* 2010;27(3):244-8.

[21] Ulanova VI, Zinzerling VA. Clinical and morphological characteristics of infective endocarditis in HIV-infected drug addicts. *Arkhiv Patologii* 2006;68(3):14-8.

[22] Zaitsev VS, Zinzerling VA, Tsvetkov EA. Clinicomorphological characteristics of laryngeal papillomatosis in children. *Arkhiv Patologii* 2005;67(2):27-9.

[23] Chumakova MA, Chumakova TG, Chumakov AA. Cavernous hemangiomas of the skin of the face and neck and the oral soft tissues. *Arkhiv Patologii.* 2007;69(5):41-4.

[24] Paltsev MA, Anichkov NM. *Patologicheskaya Anatomia* [*Pathological anatomy*] Moscow: Medicina, 2001.

[25] Frank GA, Kaplanskaia IB, Glasko EN, Semenov EA, Roshchina LS, Korolev AV. Diagnosis of lymphoproliferative diseases by bone marrow trepanobiopsy specimens. *Arkhiv Patologii* 2007;69(3):15-8.

[26] Chazov EI, Tertov VV, Orekhov AN, Lyakishev AA, Perova NV, Kurdanov KA, Khashimov KA, Novikov ID, Smirnov VN. Atherogenicity of blood serum from patients with coronary heart disease. *Lancet* 1986;2(8507):595-8.

[27] Jargin SV. Development of antiatherosclerotic drugs on the basis of cell models. *Int J Pharmacol Phytochem Ethnomed* 2015;1:10-14.

Chapter 10

INVASIVE PROCEDURES WITH QUESTIONABLE INDICATIONS

ABSTRACT

This chapter summarizes several preceding papers on invasive procedures applied with questionable clinical indications in the former Soviet Union: mastectomy with the removal of muscles, cauterization of endocervical ectopies independently of the presence of epithelial dysplasia, parabulbar injections of placebos, questionable surgical treatments of gastroduodenal ulcers, diabetes mellitus and bronchial asthma, overuse of endoscopic methods, manual therapy of the cervical spine, some questionable strategies applied in alcoholism and COVID-19. Among factors contributing to the continued use of some invasive procedures with unproven efficiency have been partial isolation from the international scientific community, disregard of the principles of informed consent and scientific polemics. It is known that invasive procedures can exert a placebo effect. However, placebo must be harmless by definition; in case of potential adverse effects it is called pseudoplacebo.

INTRODUCTION

This chapter summarizes several preceding papers on invasive procedures applied with questionable clinical indications in the former Soviet Union (SU) [1-3]. According to the author's estimates following his practice abroad, an average size of malignant tumors in surgical specimens was larger in Russia than in West Europe. Obviously, it reflects the efficiency of cancer diagnostics [4, 5]. Outside of the former SU, almost all mastectomy specimens were without muscle. The worldwide tendency towards more conservative breast cancer treatment remained unnoticed in the former SU for some period. The modified radical mastectomy of Patey with the removal of pectoralis minor muscle has been a standard treatment until recently; but the Halsted procedure with the removal of both pectoralis muscles was applied as well. In the 1980s and decreasingly during the 1990s, the Halsted operation was the widespread method of breast cancer management [6]; it was presented as the main treatment modality for breast cancer in some textbooks edited after the year 2000 [7]. Mastectomy methods with the removal of pectoralis minor muscle have been patented [8, 9].

The cauterization or cryodestruction of endocervical ectopies (pseudo-erosions) independently of the presence of epithelial dysplasia were applied routinely. Ectopies were detected at mass examinations and treated by coagulation; more details and references are in [1]. This disagrees with the international practice and is not protective against cervical cancer [10]. In particular, the recommended treatment of large ectropions by diathermoconization was noticed to cause complications [11]. Destructive treatment methods of endocervical ectopies have been patented recently [12-14]. At the same time, Pap-smears have been rare and technically suboptimal, cervical cancer being detected averagely late [15]. Even if a Pap-smear or cervical biopsy was performed, it did not always prevent the overtreatment, the more so as the difference between the terms metaplasia and dysplasia has not been uniformly understood. Pathologists were discouraged from using the term 'metaplasia' to prevent overtreatment, remittance of patients to oncological institutions (dispensaries) etc. It should be commented that the occurrence of single-layered columnar epithelium beyond the external cervical orifice i.e., endocervical ectopy is generally considered normal especially if the hormonal contraception is used.

The parabulbar and subconjunctival injections of carcinine, taurine and mildronate used in age-related vascular ophthalmic conditions [16, 17], seen to be complicated by hematomas, have been commented previously [18]. The effect of mildronate - if any - could have been adverse due to the diminished availability of adenosine triphosphate as the energy carrier [19]. A benefit from a short-term enrichment of these substances in orbital tissues can hardly be understood, while parabulbar injections are associated with risk. The same pertains to the parabulbar injections of polypeptides extracted from bovine retina (Retinalamin), other allogeneic substances and antioxidants [20-22]. Injections of cells obtained from abortion specimens into coronary vessels in dilated cardiomyopathy [23, 24] have been commented previously [25]. In conditions of suboptimal procedural quality assurance, endoscopic and endovascular manipulations can lead to infectious and thrombotic complications.

Diabetes Mellitus

The “pancreatic blood shunting into the systemic blood flow” was recommended and applied as a surgical treatment method for moderate to severe insulin-dependent diabetes mellitus [26]. The same surgery was used also in type 2 diabetes [27, 28]. The physiological rationale sounds doubtfully: “Creating a more optimal interaction of subcutaneously administered insulin and pancreas-secreted glucagon” [29]. Among 415 patients, early post-operative complications were observed in 28 ones including 2 cases of sepsis, ileus (1 cases), pyelonephritis (5 cases), pneumonia (5 cases); 2 patients died during the first week post-surgery. Ketonuria was observed in 18 cases [26] agreeing with the known fact that surgical stress can provoke ketosis in diabetics. Comparable percentages of complications were reported in [29]. The patients were subdivided into groups with a good, satisfactory and absent effect [30]. As there was no group with complications or worsening, the results must have been biased. Apart from several publications from Russia and Ukraine [26-33], no reports on this treatment of diabetes were found. Thrombosis of the splenorenal anastomosis was found angiographically in 27% of patients during eight months post-surgery [31]. Thrombosis and peritoneal adhesions were observed, while severe acidosis was a typical occurrence [31, 32]. The anti-diabetic effect of the shunting was reported to be moderate both in humans and in preceded experiments with dogs. In the experiment, the majority of dogs did not survive the induction of diabetes by streptozotocin or pancreatic resection with subsequent shunting surgery [34].

The porto-systemic shunting in diabetes was recently presented as an important achievement [35]. By 2010, the procedure was still in use while a "high thrombus-related hazard" was pointed out [32]. At the surgery, wedge biopsies from the pancreas and kidney were collected. The histological descriptions included glomerulitis with mesangial interposition, displacement of mesangial cells to the periphery of capillary loops, double-contoured glomerular basement membranes and mesangiolysis, presented as typical features and consecutive phases of diabetic glomerulosclerosis [36]; more details and references are in Chapter 11. These features are in fact characteristic of membranoproliferative glomerulonephritis which, if found in a diabetic patient, should be interpreted as a superimposed condition. The renal biopsy is generally indicated for diabetics only if a renal condition other than diabetic nephropathy is suspected. The positioning of morphological features of glomerulonephritis as characteristics of diabetic nephropathy is misleading. Moreover, renal and pancreatic biopsies are associated with risks. The same can be said about renal and splenic venography, celiac arteriography and other invasive procedures performed within the framework of the diabetes treatment by the same scientists [29].

Gastroduodenal Ulcers

Some approaches to the surgical treatment of gastroduodenal ulcers in the former SU have been different from the international practice [37]. According to the author's observations, resection of the stomach (gastrectomy) was rarely performed abroad for peptic ulcers, the volume was smaller, usually corresponding to the antrectomy. For perforated ulcers, a local excision was usually performed in Europe; and a ring-shaped specimen was sent for histological examination. In the former SU, a primary gastrectomy (2/3-3/4 of the stomach), antrectomy with vagotomy, or a simple suture (depending on the patient's condition) have usually been performed [38-41]. It was reported in 2014 that a simple closure was performed in 80% of ulcer perforations in Russia [42].

The limited availability of modern medical therapy was referred to as a "social indication" for gastrectomy for peptic ulcers [40]. During the 1960-1970s, when gastrectomy was virtually the only available surgical treatment of peptic ulcers [43], complications were noticed [37]. The hyper-radicalism in gastric surgery originates from the well-known surgeon Sergei Yudin (1891-1954). Yudin's works recommending gastrectomy for ulcers were reprinted with approving comments [44]. Yudin's authority is alive; his works continue to be cited [45, 46]. The partial gastrectomy has been advocated for perforated ulcers by many experts [37, 40, 47-51]. The broad acceptance of this procedure has been ascribed to the conservatism, non-compliance of patients and limited availability of modern medical therapy of peptic ulcers [37, 40]. In some papers advocating gastrectomy (stomach resection) for peptic ulcers, it was suggested that the "modern medical treatment does not completely solve the problem" [51] and "…does not lead to a complete recovery", so that surgery should be implemented early enough to prevent complications [48]. This approach is generally at variance with the international practice [52].

RESPIRATORY DISEASES

Another surgical procedure with no analogy in the contemporary international practice is the thoracotomy with the lung denervation in bronchial asthma [53-56] referred to as "the most recognized method" in the guidelines by the Ministry of Health [54]. The denervation was applied because it supposedly "interrupts pathological impulses from the nervous system" [53]. This argumentation was usual in the literature from the Soviet period, where so-called ideas of nervism, based on the concept of the trophic function of nervous system developed by Ivan Pavlov (1849-1936), were propagated. In particular, histological descriptions of "dystrophy" or degeneration of neural structures e.g., ganglia of the autonomic nervous system were presented as a reason for the surgical denervation [53]. The procedure was recommended by the Health Ministry while thoracotomy with the pulmonary root skeletonization was called "the most recognized surgical procedure to treat severe asthma" [54]. The pulmonary root skeletonization method was patented [57] and recommended both for "infectious-allergic" and steroid-dependent asthma [54]. Lung denervation, segment- and lobectomies were advocated even for those asthma patients in whom the medical treatment "had a temporary effect", especially in the presence of focal inflammation in the lungs. It was pointed out that the medical therapy before the surgery should be of limited duration [54]. One group of experts performed denervation procedures in 457 asthmatics. Among them, the following complications were observed: inflammation in general (27 cases), pneumonia, empyema, pneumothorax (11 cases), dysphagia, vocal fold palsy, Horner syndrome (12 cases), paraplegia, hemiparesis (2 cases); post-operative complications in general (58 cases); 6 patients died within 32 days post-surgery [56]. By 2002, the method was still in use [55]. The denervation surgery was sometimes combined with a resection of pathologically altered (from the surgeons' viewpoint) pulmonary segments or lobes [54]. Histological descriptions of surgical specimens were often trivial: inflammation and fibrosis without specifying the extension and severity. Segment- and lobectomies were applied as an independent method of the asthma treatment, even in those cases when medical therapy was effective. Indications for the surgical treatment included local pulmonary lesions such as bronchiectasis, pneumocirrhosis and bronchitis deformans (the two latter terms are used in Russia) [58]. Resections were performed also when the lesions had been extensive or bilateral, thus being not completely removable. The surgery was performed also in remissions, deemed necessary for a radical healing of asthma. This concept was advocated by Fedor Uglov [58, 59], who declared the "removal of the infectious focus" to be the main purpose of the asthma surgery. Chronic pneumonia was claimed to be "the basis of bronchial asthma" [58]. Asthmatics were transferred from therapeutic departments for the surgical and bronchoscopic treatment [59]. "After a course of therapeutic Bs", Uglov and co-workers [58] performed segment- and lobectomies, removing pulmonary tissues regarded by them to be abnormal, as a treatment method of asthma and chronic pneumonia. The same procedures were applied in various institutions also to children with persistent cough and recurrent pneumonias. Malformations alternating with intact pulmonary tissues were described histologically in the surgical specimens [60, 61]. Some descriptions of supposed malformations deviated from those in the standard editions of pulmonary pathology, being apparently adapted to the concept of surgical treatment.

ENDOSCOPY

The use of endoscopy with questionable indications has been discussed previously [2]. The broadening of indications for bronchoscopy (Bs) was associated with the names of Fedor Uglov and Lev Ioffe. Ioffe claimed that "Bs must be performed in all pulmonary diseases" [62, 63]. Uglov reported on ~6000 Bs performed in children and adults with chronic pneumonia, bronchitis and bronchial asthma with the purpose of "assessment of inflammatory changes in the bronchial tree" [59]. He maintained that Bs is indicated for diagnostics of almost all respiratory diseases also at early stages. The "complete bronchological examination" of asthmatics was regarded to be necessary. Thousands of Bs in children and adults were performed also in peripheral hospitals and outpatient centers. At the same time, difficulties of local anesthesia were noticed, which necessitated a repeated procedure under the general anesthesia in 20-25% of cases [64]. After a course of therapeutic Bs, resections of pulmonary segments or lobes deemed irreversibly changed were performed [65, 66]. Bs was recommended for asthmatics during both remissions and exacerbations, including "pre-asthma" defined as bronchitis with "elements" of bronchospasm and allergy [65, 66]. Bs was discussed as a method of early diagnostics for all forms of bronchial asthma; it was applied repeatedly for the purpose of monitoring [65]. Bs with bronchial biopsy was performed in asthmatics also for the purpose of research, sometimes repeatedly, in mild and moderate cases, both in children and the elderly [66, 67]. In parallel, Bs in asthma was noticed to be associated with the enhanced complication rate. The same experts performed 388 Bs in 216 asthmatics entailing no changes of the diagnoses [68]. Furthermore, bronchoscopic laser treatment was applied in asthma and bronchitis, also in cases with atrophy of bronchial mucosa, atrophic bronchitis and primary atrophic bronchopathy [69, 70]. Atrophic tissues are vulnerable. It is known that laser causes heating at lower absorbed energies and damage at higher energies. Both flexible and rigid bronchoscopes were used [71]. In pediatric acute pneumonia, Bs was performed to determine the type of inflammation: catarrhal vs. purulent. In patients with chronic pneumonia it was also used to exclude tuberculosis and congenital malformations [72]. Bs was applied in bronchitis, acute and chronic pneumonia, also for research [73-76], including community-acquired pneumonia (1478 procedures in 977 young patients) [77]. Bs and gastrodoudenoscopy were used as a second line screening in asthma and bronchitis diagnosed in ~4% of children "from ecologically disadvantaged areas" [78]. Endoscopic monitoring was applied in tuberculosis also with non-specific bronchial lesions [79]. Bs has been used as a second line screening method for tuberculosis in children [80].

Bronchial biopsy specimens were used for research, although the quality of histological images was sometimes suboptimal [2, 81].

Histological descriptions were often stereotype, while morphometric and other quantitative values tended to change according to the concept; more references and images are in [2]. Some histological descriptions were dubious e.g., progressive atrophy of bronchial mucosa in asthmatic children, or subatrophy found in ~80% of asthmatic children ≥12 years old [71]. In some bronchial biopsy studies, scanning electron microscopy was the only morphological method used [73], being probably irrelevant for the diagnosis. Biopsies were taken for research from large bronchi of patients with confirmed lung cancer, while the quality of histological and electron-microscopic specimens was inadequate [2, 81]. Another example: lavage fluid from patients with lung cancer or tuberculosis (also with circumscribed lesions such as tuberculoma) was used for research by infrared spectroscopy with no consequences for the therapy [82]. Gastrodoudenoscopy with biopsies for research was applied in children and adults with rheumatoid arthritis, dermatomyositis, scleroderma, systemic lupus erythematosus, uremia, various respiratory and hepatobiliary conditions, as well as for the screening of children born to asthmatic mothers [62, 78, 83-87].

MANUAL THERAPY

Various methods of manual therapy, kinesiatrics and combined programs are used in osteoarthritis (OA), other joint and spine diseases. According to systematic reviews, the manual therapy, exercise and their combinations provide relief for unspecific neck pain at least in the short-term [88, 89]. However, the role of placebo-effect is sometimes difficult to assess [90]. Undoubtedly, the patients' perception of outcome is important, especially for the assessment of subjective symptoms, disability and quality of life [91]. However, a physical treatment should not be excessive. In particular, caution must be expressed in regard to manual therapy of conditions with degenerative changes and insufficient regeneration: OA, spine lesions e.g., after professional activities such as the heavy weight bearing, those with vertebrobasilar insufficiency [92], symptoms of "severe compressive vascular vertebral syndromes" [93], functional compromise of the vertebral artery or "vertebral artery syndrome" [94] and chronic pain [95]. More examples: manual therapy of osteochondrosis (the term was used within the meaning of OA) by the pressure with therapist's thumbs up to the sensation of pain in the C1-C7 area, back- and sideward (up to 60° from vertical) movements and turning (up to 90°) of the patient's head [96]; manual therapy of "cervical spondyloarthritis aggravated by vertigo" by pushing with the therapist's knuckles (10-12 kg/cm^2, multiple courses) [97]. Adverse events following manual treatments to the spine are common, although serious complications are rare [98-100]. In particular, cervical spine manipulations may carry a small risk for neurovascular complications [101-103]. There is an opinion that the non-superiority to other treatments, coupled with concerns regarding safety, renders cervical spine manipulations inadvisable [101]. Certainly, the maintenance of an optimum level of the physical fitness is important; but the balance between the exercise and rest should be reasonable especially in degenerative diseases, wear and tear conditions in aged people as well as certain posttraumatic lesions. For example, it is often stated that the hand exercises in OA should be of low intensity, performed in periods with little pain and inflammation. It is not surprising that splints i.e., immobilization reduced hand pain in OA more consistently than exercises. A meta-analysis demonstrated that splints significantly reduced the hand pain [104]. Obviously, in conditions of insufficient regeneration, cartilaginous structures should be protected from further damage.

Alcoholism and Alcoholics

The following treatments were applied to alcoholics: prolonged intravenous infusions, sorbent hemoperfusion, endolymphatic and endobronchial drug delivery, pyrotherapy with sulfozine (oil solution of sulphur for intramuscular injections), endoscopic and surgical biopsies of internal organs, endoscopic cholangiopancreatography and angiography without clear indications also for research [105, 106]; more details and references are in [3, 107]. The differential diagnosis of hangover vs. alcohol withdrawal syndrome is a known problem [108]; it is of particular importance for Russia, where these conditions are not clearly distinguished from each other in some handbooks and official instructions. Although combinations are possible, the hangover is different from the alcohol withdrawal syndrome, the latter being largely a result of neuroadaptation after a long-term consumption [109]. The detoxification by intravenous infusions of sodium chloride, dextran, magnesium (Mg) sulphate, glucose solutions etc. have been recommended for various forms of alcohol dependence and alcoholism including the "moderately severe withdrawal syndrome" [110-113]. This is at variance with the international literature. Alcohol and its derivatives are eliminated spontaneously while rehydration can be usually achieved per os. Intravenous glucose and Mg are generally not recommended in the settings of alcohol withdrawal syndrome [114, 115]. Excessive infusions of Mg-containing solutions are associated with adverse effects observed also in treated alcoholics [113, 116]. Repeated intravenous manipulations are associated with risks and discomfort especially for patients with narrow, collapsed veins. Especially in conditions of suboptimal procedural quality assurance, endovascular and endoscopic manipulations can lead to the transmission of viral hepatitis, which occurred to treated alcoholic patients. A combination of the viral and alcoholic liver injury is known to be unfavorable. Compulsory treatments of alcoholics with tuberculosis included repeated Bs. Among others, vocal cord injuries were observed in such patients; more details are in [2]. Furthermore, it was noticed that vigorous apomorphine- and mechanically induced vomiting as emetic (aversive) therapy of alcohol dependence induced bleeding in some patients with pulmonary tuberculosis [117]. It was reported in 1994 that about 60% of patients of a "phtisio-narcological" institution for the compulsory treatment escaped while a half of them was returned with the help of the police (militia) [118].

The ultra-rapid (one session) treatment of alcoholism, known in the former SU as 'coding', should be commented briefly. This method was started during the anti-alcohol campaign; it was regarded to be incompatible with medical ethics because of mystification, verbal intimidation and painful manipulations associated with health risks. The following has been applied: spraying of the throat or infusion of 3-5 ml ethyl chloride into the pharynx with enforced swallowing, intensive pressure with therapist's thumbs on the trigeminal and greater occipital nerve branches, pressure on the carotid sinus areas or the patient's eyeballs, intralingual injections, turning and forceful backwards movements of the patient's head [119-126]. The latter manipulation is associated with a risk of injury especially for patients with vertebral abnormalities.

COVID-19

The following citations from the Recommendations on COVID-19 issued by the Ministry of Heath should be commented (verbatim from Russian): "Indications to the tracheal intubation (one of the following criteria suffices): hypoxemia with the oxygen saturation according to pulse oximetry $SpO_2 < 92\%$ despite the high flow oxygen delivery in the prone position; respiratory rate >35 breaths per minute; increase in the visible thorax excursions; derangements of consciousness; deterioration of the X-ray picture of the lungs; apnea; unstable hemodynamics" [127]. Moreover, the intubation is indicated at SpO_2 = 90-92%, respiratory rate >26, combined with symptoms such as agitation and anxiety [127]. According to the recommendations, a patient testing positive for COVID-19 must be hospitalized in the presence of one of the following criteria: respiratory rate ≥ 22; $SpO_2 < 93\%$; mild course of the disease in a patient >65 years old or in combination with diabetes mellitus, chronic heart failure or a respiratory disease (bronchial asthma, chronic obstructive pulmonary disease) etc. [127]. Obviously, hospitalization is associated with stress, risks of nosocomial infections and iatrogenic adverse events especially for aged people. One of the motives of the over-manipulation may be the personnel training, which pertains also to some other invasive methods with questionable indications discussed here. Apparently, similar considerations are also relevant to China, where some literature advises against non-invasive ventilation methods: "Debate exists regarding the use of high-flow nasal oxygen therapies or noninvasive ventilation for concerns of aerosolization of the virus, so it is commonly not recommended [128]. Therefore, these authors and many others have come to a reasonable conclusion that it is best to intubate earlier in the disease progression. The authors also observed a high rate of pneumothorax (5.9%) after intubation" [129]. In the above-cited article [128] it is written: "If manual bagging is required, we suggest gentle ventilation via a supraglottic device instead of bag mask ventilation." The main reason of these recommendations is the concern about the staff safety because non-invasive ventilation is supposedly associated with the virus aerosolization [128, 129]. Of note, both endotracheal tube and supraglottic (laryngeal mask airway) ventilation is associated with adverse effects [130]. Prioritizing the personnel's safety over that of patients is contradictory to the principle "Primum non nocere" (first do no harm). Note that critically ill patients are averagely much older than the staff thus undergoing higher risks; it would be obviously against the medical ethics to decide in favor of an intubation or another invasive method to protect caregivers. Initial suggestions for early intubation of COVID-19 patients may have caused harm [131]. To prevent the overtreatment, it should be stressed that the basic airway management principles apply to known or suspected COVID-19 cases, as they do with other critically ill patients [132]. With regard to infectious aerosols, better ventilation of rooms substantially reduces the airborne time of respiratory droplets, which is important for hospital settings where the aerosolization by coughing and medical treatments is common [133]. The course of the disease and the possibility of intubation must be discussed with patients possibly early (optimally on admission), so that they could make an informed decision about the possibility to undergo intubation and mechanical ventilation [134].

Some health workers' rights can be violated during pandemic [135] e.g., the principle of informed consent to invasive procedures. Medical personnel in Russia obligatorily undergoes regular (once in 7-10 days) SARS-CoV-2 antibody tests using venous blood. Repeated intravenous manipulations are associated with risks and discomfort especially for patients with narrow, collapsed veins. If the antibody test is positive, both nasal and pharyngeal swabs are taken for the PCR-based assay, also from known convalescents and persons with the positive viral tests in the past who thereafter have tested negatively twice i.e., after a negative seroconversion. The smears may be taken with urogenital swabs using excessive force. Mucosal damage might predispose to infections. Nasal swabs are taken also from persons with atrophic rhinitis, a history of nasal bleedings, septum ulcerations etc. An inquiry directed to the health care authority was replied with a reference to the instructive Letter Nr. 02-706-2020-27 of 21 January 2020 issued by the Federal Service for Surveillance on Consumer Rights Protection and Human Wellbeing (Rospotrebnadzor) that swabs from the nasal cavity and nasopharynx are obligatory. Indeed, there are no specific contraindications for collecting specimens with nasopharyngeal swabs. However, clinicians should be cautious if the patient has had recent nasal trauma or surgery, has a markedly deviated nasal septum, a history of chronically blocked nasal passages or severe coagulopathy [136]. When collection of a nasopharyngeal swab is not possible, the following are acceptable alternatives: an oropharyngeal specimen, a nasal mid-turbinate specimen (using a flocked tapered swab), an anterior nares specimen (using a flocked or spun polyester swab), a nasopharyngeal wash/aspirate or nasal aspirate specimen [137].

Serologic antibody tests can reveal those individuals who were infected and didn't know it. However, for known convalescents and/or those after a negative seroconversion, the repeated serological tests seem to be useless. If a person is serologically found immune, it is unlikely that he or she would get reinfected [138]. In fact, the antibody testing can be used to return people with immunity to the workforce or keep them there, starting with health care professionals. "A positive antibody test could be a sort of get-out-of-isolation card" [138]. Admittedly, there is not enough evidence to conclude that the detection of SARS-CoV-2-specific antibodies can be linked to the end of the viral infectivity [139]. More details are in [140].

CONCLUSION

It is known that the concept of informed consent has not been uniformly accepted in Russia. Today, patients are sometimes requested to sign in advance a form certifying their blanket consent to unnamed diagnostic and therapeutic procedures. In regard to the endoscopy, informed consent has been mentioned only in some recent papers. For asthmatic children aged 5-15 years, the consent of parents was regarded to be sufficient for participation in a bronchoscopic study [141]. Note that the principles of informed consent or assent are applicable also to children and adolescents [142, 143]. Factors contributing to the persistence of suboptimal methods included the partial isolation from the international scientific community, authoritative management style, disapproval of criticism, oblivion of the rules of scientific polemics, insufficient use of the foreign literature and unavailability of many internationally used handbooks even in central medical libraries [144, 145]. Disregard for the principles of informed consent together with authoritative and paternalistic attitudes towards patients contributed to the use of invasive methods with questionable indications. Today, the Russian-language literature is increasingly aware of foreign publications, while the practice is being adjusted to international standards. However, some papers containing questionable recommendations have remained without due commentaries, so that the possibility of reversion to suboptimal practices is not excluded today. The placebo effect exerted by some invasive treatments is a recognized occurrence. However, placebo must be harmless by definition; in case of adverse effects it is designated as pseudoplacebo [146].

REFERENCES

[1] Jargin SV. Surgical procedures with questionable indications: A letter from Russia. *J Surgery* 2016;4(1):6.

[2] Jargin SV. On the endoscopic methods used with questionable indications. *J Surgery* 2016;4:6.

[3] Jargin SV. Some aspects of renal biopsy for research. *Int J Nephrol Kidney Failure* 2015;1:1-5.

[4] Jargin S. *Thyroid cancer after Chernobyl: Re-evaluation needed. Turk Patoloji Derg* 2020; doi:10.5146/tjpath.2020.01489.

[5] Jargin SV. Post-Chernobyl renal cancers vs. control from Spain and Colombia: A comment. *J Oncology* 2020;1(1):1002.

[6] Semiglazov VF, Volkov ON, Semiglazov VV. *The problem of breast cancer on the eve of 21th century.* Saint Petersburg, Medical University, 1998.

[7] Semiglazov VV, Topuzov EE. *Breast cancer.* Moscow: Medpress-inform, 2009.

[8] Druzhkov BK, Druzhkov OB. *The method of extended mastectomy.* Patent RU95106525A1 (1995).

[9] Tsejlikman EG, Patsyrova LA, Vaganov. NV. *Method of mastectomy with preservation of greater pectoral muscle.* Patent RU2335249C2 (2008).

[10] Machado Jr LC, Dalmaso AS, Carvalho HB. Evidence for benefits from treating cervical ectopy: literature review. *Sao Paulo Med J* 2008;126:132-9.

[11] Bychkov VI, Bykov EG, Bratus AM. Complications and late results of the treatment of precancerous conditions of the cervix uteri by diathermic conization. *Akush Ginekol* (Mosk) 1990;(2);61-62.

[12] Zubkovskaja EV, Lipatov IS, Tezikov, JV, Bljumina IZ. *Way of treatment of pseudo-erosion of uterine neck.* Patent RU2361632C2 (2009).

[13] Kochenov VI, Vaganova SE, Tsybusov SN. *Method for applying cryogenic therapy to treat uterine cervix diseases.* Patent RU2291673C1 (2007).

[14] Khvorostukhina NF, Novichkov DA, Mikheeva JV, Stoljarova UV, Stepanova N.N. *Method of treating cervical ectopia.* Patent RU2568768C1 (2015).

[15] Jargin SV. Perspectives of cervical cytology in Russia. *Am J Obstet Gynecol* 2008;199(2):e10.
[16] Solomatin II. Use of the mildronate preparation in ophthalmology. In: *VI Forum Ophtalmologicum Balticum.* Riga: LMA, 1990; 97-99.
[17] Shpak NI, Naritsyna NI, Konovalova NV. Taufon and emoksipin in the combined treatment of sclerotic macular dystrophies. *Oftalmol Zh* 1989;(7):463-5.
[18] Jargin SV. On the use of carnosine and antioxidants. *J Intercult Ethnopharmacol 2016*;5:317-19.
[19] Jargin SV. Meldonium (Mildronate): Primum non nocere. *Pharmacol Res* 2016;114:294.
[20] Lastochkina EK, Chekhova TA. *Method for treatment of vascular and dystrophic ophthalmopathies.* Patent RU2367388C1 (2009).
[21] Ljalin AN, Zharov VV, Butolina OE. *Method of treating involutional eye diseases.* Patent RU2565840C2 (2015).
[22] Mirkhaidarov RSh, Urazbakhtin RK, Mirkhaidarova ZM, Ruchko A.Iu. *Treatment method of eye diseases by parabulbar injections of dispersed Alloplant biomaterial.* Patent RU2016130029A (2018).
[23] Fatkhutdinov TKh, D'yachkov AV, Koroteyev AV, Goldstein DV, Bochkov NP. Safety and efficiency of transplantation of allogenic multipotent stromal cells in surgical treatment of dilatated cardiomyopathy. *Bull Exp Biol Med* 2010;149:119-24.
[24] Gol'dshtejn DV, Makarov AV, Volkov AV, Fatkhudinov TK, Rzhaninova AA. et al. *Biotransplant and method for treating chronic cardiac failure (variants).* Patent RU2299073C1 (2007).
[25] Jargin SV. Stem cells and cell therapies in cardiology. *International Journal of Cardiology Research* 2019;1(1):10-12.
[26] Diuzheva TG. *Surgical treatment of patients with insulindependent diabetes mellitus.* Dissertation. Moscow: Sechenov Medical Academy, 1992.
[27] Putintsev AM, Shraer TI, Sergeev VN, Maslov MG, Strukova OA. Variants of surgical management for severe arterial hypertension combined with type 2 diabetes mellitus. *Angiol Sosud Khir* 2010;16(2):120-5.

[28] Kirnus LM, Che V, Makarov NA, Burovkin BA, Shvartsshtejn VJa. et al. Method for surgically treating the cases of second type diabetes mellitus. Patent RU2036610C1 (1995).

[29] Galperin EI, Diuzheva TG, Petrovsky PF, Chevokin AYu, Dokuchayev KV, et al. Results of pancreatic blood shunting into the systemic blood flow in insulin-dependent diabetics. *HPB Surg* 1996;9:191-7.

[30] Galperin EI, Diuzheva TG, Rabinovich SE, Platonova LV, Severgina ES, et al. Distal spleno-renal shunt. A surgical approach to the management of diabetes mellitus patients. *Annals of Surgical Hepatolog.* 1996;1:77-90.

[31] Nikonenko AS, Kovalev AA, Zavgorodnii SN, Volkova NA. Surgical treatment of insulin-dependent diabetes mellitus and its complications. *Khirurgiia* (Mosk) 1996;(2):81-83.

[32] Torgunakov SA, Torgunakov AP. Possible causes of thrombusrelated hazard of a distal splenorenal venous anasto-mosis. *Angiol Sosud Khir* 2010;16(4):184-8.

[33] Torgunakov AP, Torgunakov SA, Magerramova E.F. *Method for surgical treatment of diabetes mellitus.* Patent RU2421163C1 (2011).

[34] Gal'perin EI, Kuzovlev NF, Diuzheva TG, Aleksandrovskaia TN. Approaches to surgical treatment of diabetes mellitus (experimental study). *Khirurgiia* (Mosk) 1983;(1):13-20.

[35] Editorial. Galperin E.I. 80th anniversary. *Khirurgiia* (Mosk) 2011;(8):103-4.

[36] Severgina ES, Ponomarev AB, Diuzheva TG, Shestakova MV, Maiorova EM (1994) Diabetic glomerulonephritis - the first stage of diabetic glomerulopathy. *Arkh Patol* 56: 44-50.

[37] Balalykin DA. Introduction of pathogenic principles of surgical treatment of ulcer disease in Russian surgery. *Khirurgiia* (Mosk) 2004;(10):73-78.

[38] Afendulov SA, Zhuravlev GIu, Smirnov AD, Krasnolutskii NA. Preventive surgical treatment of ulcer disease. *Vestn Khir Im I I Grek* 2006;165(3):18-23.

[39] Potashov LV, Semenov DIu, Ushveridze DG, Osmanov ZKh, Chekmasov IuS, et al. Long-term results of closure of perforated pyloro-duodenal ulcers. *Vestn Khir Im I I Grek* 2005;164(5):40-42.

[40] Gostishchev VK, Evseev MA, Golovin RA. Radical operative treatment of perforative gastroduodenal ulcer disease. *Khirurgiia* (Mosk) 2009;(3):10-16.

[41] Vachev AN, Koryttsev VK, Antropov IV. *Method of selecting operation volume in case of perforated ulcers of stomach and duodenum.* Patent RU2506886C1 (2014).

[42] Sazhin IV, Sazhin VP, Bronshtein PG, Savel'ev VM, Nuzhdikhin AV, et al. Laparoscopic treatment of perforated ulcers. *Khirurgiia* (Mosk) 2014;(7):12-16.

[43] Pantsyrev IuM, Mikhalev AI, Fedorov ED, Cherniakevich SA. Surgical treatment of complicated ulcer disease. In: Saveliev VS (eds) *Eighty lectures in surgery.* Moscow: Litterra, 2008.

[44] Iudin SS. Essays on gastric surgery. *Khirurgiia* (Mosk) 1991; (7):159-66.

[45] Abakumov MM, Kuzibayeva MP. The letters from the exile of the academician S.S. Yudin. *Khirurgiia* (Mosk) 2012;(4):81-85.

[46] Nishanov FN, Batirov AK, Abdiraiimov BA, Abdullazhanov BR, Nishanov MF. Current state of the problem of surgical treatment of perforating duodenal ulcers. *Vestn Khir Im I I Grek* 2011;170(5):97-100.

[47] Kuzin MI, Chistova MA. *The stomach and duodenum. In: Kuzin MA, editor. Surgical diseases*. Moscow: Meditsina, 1995; 337-407.

[48] Babalich AK. Surgical treatment of patients with duodenal ulcer. *Khirurgiia* (Mosk) 1999;(7):19-22.

[49] Vachev AN, Korytsev VK, Antropov IV. The choice of resection volume by the combination of perforative duodenal ulcer with other complications of the ulcer disease. *Khirurgiia* (Mosk) 2013;(11):29-31.

[50] Repin VN, Kostylev LM, Poliakov SN, Matveeva NA. Choice of the operation for perforated ulcers of the stomach and duodenum. *Vestn Khir Im I I Grek* 2011;170(2):48-51.

[51] Komarov NV, Maslagin AS, Komarov RN. Surgical treatment of patients with complications of peptic ulcer of the stomach and duodenum under conditions of a regional hospital. *Vestn Khir Im I I Grek* 2001;160(2):104-6.

[52] Chung KT, Shelat VG. Perforated peptic ulcer - an update. *World J Gastrointest Surg* 2017;9:1-12.

[53] Babichev SI, Kharlampovich SI, Tarasova LB, Smakov GM, Savchenko ZI. Partial denervation of the lungs in bronchial asthma. *Khirurgiia* (Mosk) 1985;(4):31-35.

[54] Health Ministry of RSFSR. *Indications and contraindications for the surgical treatment of bronchial asthma.* Moscow, 1988.

[55] Gudovskii LM, Karashurov SE, Karashurov ES, Volkov AA, Parshin VD. Surgical treatment of bronchial asthma. *Khirurgiia* (Mosk) 2002;(7):14-18.

[56] Smakov GM. Complications of surgical treatment of patients with bronchial asthma. *Khirurgiia* (Mosk) 1990;(2):124-7.

[57] Giller BM, Giller DB, Giller GV. *Method for surgical treatment of bronchial asthma.* Patent RU2074645C1 (1997).

[58] Uglov FG. *Pathogenesis, clinic and therapy of chronic pneumonia.* Moscow: Meditsina, 1976.

[59] Uglov FG. *Under the white mantle.* Moscow, Sovietskaia Rossia, 1984.

[60] Esipova IK, Vladimirtseva AL. Congenital malformations of the lungs. *Arkh Patol* 1996;58(3):49-54.

[61] Esipova IK, Vladimirtseva AL, Biriukov VV. Branching defects and mucosal diverticulosis of the bronchi in children as factors predisposing to the development of chronic inflammatory processes in the lungs. *Arkh Patol* 1990;52:6-10.

[62] Aliev MA, Ioffe LTs, Kashkin KA, Goncharov AI, Ismagilov RZ. Role of endoscopy in the diagnosis and treatment of lesions of the digestive system in patients with uremia. *Klin Khir* 1987;(8):61-63.

[63] Ioffe LTs. *Non-tuberculosis pulmonary diseases, their diagnosis and treatment.* Alma-Ata, Znanie, 1976.

[64] Uglov FG. *Bronchological diagnostic methods of pulmonary diseases*. Leningrad, Research Inst. Pulmonol., 1971.

[65] Skopina EI. *Bronchoscopy in diagnostics and treatment of different clinical varieties of infectious-allergic bronchial asthma.* Dissertation. Saratov: Medical Institute, 1980.

[66] Nepomnyashchikh GI, Aidagulova SV, Trubnikova NV, Volkova DV, Bakarev MA. Structural modifications of the bronchial epithelium in asthma. *Bull Exp Biol Med* 2007;143(4):483-7.

[67] Grinshtein IuI, Shestovitskii VA. Severe bronchial asthma in elderly patients. *Adv Gerontol.* 2004;13:102-6.

[68] Mavritsin LE, Lifshits NA. Complications in the fiber bronchoscopy of bronchial asthma patients. *Klin Med* (Mosk) 1980;58(4):37-40.

[69] Chernekhovskaia NE. *Lasers in endoscopy*. Moscow: Medpress-inform, 2011.

[70] Nepomnyashchikh GI, Levitskii VA, Nepomnyashchikh LM, Aidagulova SV, Naumova LA, et al. Instability of bronchial epithelium in chronic pulmonary diseases. *Bull Exp Biol Med* 2000;129(4):396-9.

[71] Bogatyrev AF. Morphological features of airway mucosa in children with bronchial asthma. *Allergologiia* 2001;(3):7-11.

[72] Isaeva LA. *Pediatrics*. Moscow: Meditsina, 1994.

[73] Rannev IB. *Bronchoscopy in the treatment of patients with pneumonia.* Dissertation. Moscow: Academy of Advanced Medical Training, 2003.

[74] Fedchenko GG, Chernekhovskaia NE, Rannev IB. Radiation and endoscopic diagnosis of pneumonia. *Vestn Rentgenol Radiol* 2002;(1):21-26.

[75] Shpak OI, Rolik LV, Gomoliako IV. Morpho-endoscopy comparisons and analysis of bronchoalveolar washings in patients with chronic bronchitis. *Probl Tuberk* 1984;(12):53-57.

[76] Chernushenko EF, Belianovskaia TI, Rolik LV, Kuznetsova LV, Shpak OI. Determination of alveolar macrophage function in nonspecific lung diseases by the simultaneous estimation of

phagocytosis and acid phosphatase activity. *Zh Mikrobiol Epidemiol Immunobiol* 1984;(6):84-86.

[77] Kazantsev VA. The use of bronchological sanation for treatment of community-acquired pneumonia. In: Abstract book. 3rd Congress of European region. International Union against Tuberculosis and Lung diseases (IUATLD). *14th National Congress of Lung diseases;* 2004 June 22-26; Moscow, 2004; 361.

[78] Klimanskaia EV, Vozzhaeva FS. Combined lesions of respiratory organs and gastrointestinal tract in children from ecologically disadvantaged areas. *Ross Pediatr Zh* 2001;4:20-23.

[79] Filippov VP, Chernichenko NV. *Bronchoscopy in pulmonary diseases.* Moscow, Binom, 2014.

[80] Aksenova VA, Rozinova NN, Mokhnachevskaia AI, Kravchenko AF. *Detection of tuberculosis in children and adolescents with nonspecific pulmonary pathology in public health institutions.* Moscow, Sechenov Medical Academy, 2005.

[81] Nepomniashchikh LM, Levitskii VA, Nepomniashchikh GI, Aidagulova SV, Belov IIu, et al. Pathomorphologic and endoscopic analysis of large bronchi during lung cancer. *Biull Eksp Biol Med* 2000;129(3):347-51.

[82] Gelfond ML. *Diagnosis of tuberculosis by means of infrared spectroscopy of the bronchial lavage fluid.* Dissertation. Moscow: Research Inst Tuberculosis, 1996.

[83] Musaev SN, Novikova AV, Klimanskaia EV, Shershevskaia AIa. Clinico-endoscopic and morphometric characteristics of gastric and duodenal mucosa in children with dermatomyositis. *Revmatologiia* (Mosk) 1991;(4):21-25.

[84] Musaev SN, Novikova AV, Shershevskaia AIa, Klimanskaia EV, Aksenova IV. The morphometric and immunohistoche-mical characteristics of the gastric and duodenal mucosa in systemic lupus erythematosus. *Biull Eksp Biol Med* 1991;111(2):203-6.

[85] Shakhbazian IE, Garkusha MB, Sklianskaia OA, Ali NIu, Daurova NV, et al. Campylobacter pylori gastroduodenitis in children with juvenile rheumatoid arthritis. *Revmatologiia* (Mosk) 1991;(3):23-28.

[86] Tsoi EA, Balabolkin II, Geppe NA, Erdes SI. The symptoms of gastroesophageal disease from children with asthma. In: Abstract book. 3rd Congress of European region. International Union against Tuberculosis and Lung diseases (IUATLD). *14th National Congress of Lung diseases;* 2004 June 22-26; Moscow, 2004; 213.

[87] Geppe NA, Kuzmenko LE, Sazhina NA, Farobina EG. Clinical and laboratory examination of children born to mothers with bronchial asthma. In: Abstract book. 3rd Congress of European region. International Union against Tuberculosis and Lung diseases (IUATLD). *14th National Congress of Lung diseases;* 2004 June 2226; Moscow, 2004; 184.

[88] Leaver AM, Refshauge KM, Maher CG, McAuley JH. Conservative interventions provide short-term relief for non-specific neck pain: a systematic review. *J Physiother* 2010;56(2):73-85.

[89] Sterling M, de Zoete RMJ, Coppieters I, Farrell SF. Best evidence rehabilitation for chronic pain part 4: Neck pain. *J Clin Med* 2019;8(8):1219.

[90] Jargin SV. Invasive procedures with questionable indications and possible placebo effects. *Arch Clin Exp Surg* 2015;4(4):215-21.

[91] Carrasco-Uribarren A, Rodríguez-Sanz J, Hidalgo-García C, Tricás-Moreno JM, Balboa-López D, Cabanillas-Barea S. Short-term effects of an upper cervical spine traction-manipulation program in patients with cervicogenic dizziness: A case series study. *J Back Musculoskelet Rehabil* 2020; doi: 10.3233/BMR-181479.

[92] Tjan VN, Gojdenko VS. *Method of treating chronic vertebrobasilar insufficiency*. Patent RU2447876C2 (2012).

[93] Khoroshukhin VJ, Khoroshukhina OK, Tsvetkova IV. *Manual techniques applied for vertebra-neurologic syndromes.* Patent RU2325892C2 (2008).

[94] Gritsenko AG, Pavlov AB, Naziev AI, Lychkova AE. *Method for treating the cases of cervical osteochondrosis with concomitant vertebral artery syndrome.* Patent RU2150929C1 (2000).

[95] Evseev VI. *Method for treating osteochondrosis of the cervical spine*. Patent RU2654574C1 (2018).

[96] Shishonin AJu. *Method for treating cervical osteochondrosis.* Patent RU2243758C2 (2005).

[97] Gritsenko AG, Gritsenko KA. *Method for treating cervical spondyloarthritis aggravated by vertigo.* Patent RU2114595C1 (1998).

[98] Kerry R, Taylor AJ. Cervical arterial dysfunction: knowledge and reasoning for manual physical therapists. *J Orthop Sports Phys Ther* 2009;39:378-87.

[99] Swait G, Finch R. What are the risks of manual treatment of the spine? A scoping review for clinicians. *Chiropr Man Therap* 2017;25:37.

[100] Ivanenko TA. X-ray signs of ligamentous cervical injuries from joint manual therapy. *Vestn Rentgenol Radiol* 2008;(2-3):56-58.

[101] Wand BM, Heine PJ, O'Connell NE. Should we abandon cervical spine manipulation for mechanical neck pain? Yes. *BMJ* 2012;344:e3679.

[102] Hutting N, Kerry R, Coppieters MW, Scholten-Peeters GGM. Considerations to improve the safety of cervical spine manual therapy. *Musculoskelet Sci Pract* 2018;33:41-45.

[103] Hurwitz EL, Morgenstern H, Vassilaki M, Chiang LM. Frequency and clinical predictors of adverse reactions to chiropractic care in the UCLA neck pain study. *Spine* 2005;30(13):1477-84.

[104] Kjeken I, Smedslund G, Moe RH, Slatkowsky-Christensen B, Uhlig T, Hagen KB. A systematic review of design and effects of splints and exercise programs in hand osteoarthritis. *Arthritis Care Res* 2011;63:834-48.

[105] Makhov VM, Abdullin RG, Gitel' EL, Zavodnov VIa, Podzolkov VI, et al. Visceral lesions in alcoholism. *Ter Arkh* 1996;68(8):53-56.

[106] Krut'ko VS. Pneumonia in patients with pulmonary tuberculosis and alcoholism. *Probl Tuberk* 1990;(1):64-66.

[107] Jargin SV. Alcohol abuse and toxicity of alcoholic beverages in Russia: Recent history. *ARC Journal of Addiction* 2016;1(1):21-29.

[108] Boness CL, Lane SP, Sher KJ. Assessment of withdrawal and hangover is confounded in the alcohol use disorder and associated

disabilities interview schedule: Withdrawal prevalence is likely inflated. *Alcohol Clin Exp Res* 2016;40:1691-99.

[109] Boness CL, Lane SP, Sher KJ. Assessment of withdrawal and hangover is confounded in the Alcohol Use Disorder and Associated Disabilities Interview Schedule: Withdrawal prevalence is likely inflated. *Alcohol Clin Exp Res* 2016;40:1691-9.

[110] Ivanets NN, Vinnikova MA. *Alcoholism*. Moscow: MIA, 2011. (in Russsian)

[111] Shabanov PD. *Narcology*. 2nd edition. Moscow: Geotar-Media, 2015. (in Russsian)

[112] *Annex to the Order of the Health Ministry of Russian Federation* No. 140 of 28 April 1998. http://docs.cntd.ru/document/1200119087 (last accessed June 24, 2020). (in Russsian)

[113] Galankin LN, Livanov GA, Guzikov BM, et al. *The method of the tactics determination in alcohol withdrawal syndrome.* Patent RU2202946C2 (2003).

[114] Jesse S, Bråthen G, Ferrara M, et al. Alcohol withdrawal syndrome: mechanisms, manifestations, and management. *Acta Neurol Scand* 2017;135(1):4-16.

[115] Schuckit MA. Recognition and management of withdrawal delirium (delirium tremens). *N Engl J Med.* 2014;371(22):2109-13.

[116] Swaminathan R. Magnesium metabolism and its disorders. *Clin Biochem Rev* 2003;24:47-66.

[117] Entin GM (1990) *Treatment of alcoholism.* Moscow: Meditsina, Russia.

[118] Rudoi NM, Dzhokhadze VA, Chubakov TCh, Stadnikova AV. Current status and perspectives in hospital treatment of patients with tuberculosis complicated with alcohol abuse. *Probl Tuberk* 1994;(4):8-10. PMID: 7984622.

[119] Dovzhenko AR, Artemchuk AF, Bolotova ZN, Vorob'eva TM, Manuilenko IuA. Outpatient stress psychotherapy of patients with alcoholism. *Zh Nevropatol Psikhiatr Im S S Korsakova* 1988;88(2):94-97.

[120] Lipgart NK, Goloburda AV, Ivanov VV. Once more about A.R. Dobzhenko's method of stress psychotherapy in alcoholism. *Zh Nevropatol Psikhiatr Im S S Korsakova* 1991;91(6):133-4.

[121] Voskresenskii VA. Critical evaluation of ultra-rapid psychotherapy of alcoholism (concerning the article by A.R. Dovzhenko et al. "Ambulatory stress psychotherapy of alcoholics"). *Zh Nevropatol Psikhiatr Im S SKorsakova* 1990; 90:130-2.

[122] Frolov VV. *Method for treating the cases of chronic alcoholism.* Patent RU2161047C2 (2000).

[123] Dovzhenko AR, Dobrovol'skij VV, Podkova VP. *Method for treating alcoholism or/and narcotics.* Patent RU2006220C1 (1994).

[124] Kuznetsov AV, Mukhomedzjanov KhM. *Method of neurosublingual coding of alcohol dependence.* Patent RU94042546A1 (1996).

[125] Grigor'ev GG. *Method for treating alcohol, nicotine and narcotic dependence.* Patent RU2034576C1 (1996).

[126] Shorin VV. *Method to treat chronic alcoholism and/or narcomania.* Patent RU2089229C1 (1998).

[127] Kamkin EG. Vremennye metodicheskie rekomendatsii. Profilaktika, diagnostika i lechenie novoi koronavirusnoi infektsii (COVID-19) Temporary methodical recommendations. *Prevention, diagnostics and treatment of the new coronavirus infection* (COVID-19) Version 6. Moscow, Russia, Ministry of Health, April 28, 2020; pp. 55, 67, 106-7.

[128] Cheung JC, Ho LT, Cheng JV, Cham EYK, Lam KN. Staff safety during emergency airway management for COVID-19 in Hong Kong. *Lancet Respir Med* 2020;8:e19.

[129] Aziz MF. The COVID-19 intubation experience in Wuhan. *Br J Anaesth* 2020;125(1):e25-e27.

[130] Strametz R, Bergold MN, Weberschock T. Laryngeal mask airway versus endotracheal tube for percutaneous dilatational tracheostomy in critically ill adults. *Cochrane Database Syst Rev* 2018;11: CD009901.

[131] Zareifopoulos N, Lagadinou M, Karela A, Platanaki C, Karantzogiannis G, Velissaris D. Management of COVID-19: the

risks associated with treatment are clear, but the benefits remain uncertain. *Monaldi Arch Chest Dis* 2020;90:1342.

[132] Brown CA 3rd, Mosier JM, Carlson JN, Gibbs MA. Pragmatic recommendations for intubating critically ill patients with suspected COVID-19. *J Am Coll Emerg Physicians Open* 2020; doi:10.1002/emp2.12063.

[133] Somsen GA, van Rijn C, Kooij S, et al. Small droplet aerosols in poorly ventilated spaces and SARS-CoV-2 transmission. *Lancet Respir Med* 2020; doi: 10.1016/S2213-2600(20)30245-9.

[134] Zareifopoulos N, Lagadinou M, Karela A, Karantzogiannis G, Velissaris D. Intubation and mechanical ventilation of patients with COVID-19: what should we tell them? *Monaldi Arch Chest Dis.* 2020;90:1296.

[135] Sheather J, Hartwell A, Norcliffe-Brown D. Serious violations of health workers' rights during pandemic. *BMJ* 2020;370:m2824.

[136] Marty FM, Chen K, Verrill KA. How to obtain a nasopharyngeal swab specimen. *N Engl J Med* 2020;382(22):e76. doi:10.1056/NEJMvcm2010260.

[137] La Marca A, Capuzzo M, Paglia T, Roli L, Trenti T, Nelson SM. Testing for SARS-CoV-2 (COVID-19): a systematic review and clinical guide to molecular and serological in-vitro diagnostic assays. *Reprod Biomed Online* 2020; doi: 10.1016/j.rbmo.2020.06.001.

[138] Abbasi J. The promise and peril of antibody testing for COVID-19. *JAMA* 2020; doi: 10.1001/jama.2020.6170.

[139] Özçürümez MK, Ambrosch A, Frey O, et al. SARS-CoV-2 antibody testing-questions to be asked. *J Allergy Clin Immunol* 2020;146 (1):35-43.

[140] Jargin SV. COVID-19: economic damage is a health risk. *Am J Prev Med Public Health* 2020; 6(3): 62-64.

[141] Fedorov IA, Wilson SJ, Davies DE, Holgate ST. Epithelial stress and structural remodelling in childhood asthma. *Thorax* 2005;60:389-94.

[142] Neill SJ. Research with children: a critical review of the guidelines. *J Child Health Care* 2005;9:46-58.

[143] Kuther TL, Posada M. Children and adolescents' capacity to provide informed consent for participation in research. *Adv Psychol Res* 2004;32:163-73.

[144] Jargin SV. Some aspects of medical education in Russia. *Am J Med Studies* 2013;1:4-7.

[145] Murphy J, Jargin S. International trends in health science librarianship part 20: Russia. *Health Info Libr J* 2017;34:92-94.

[146] Weihrauch TR. Placebo treatment is effective differently in different diseases- but is it also harmless? A brief synopsis. *Sci Eng Ethics* 2004;10:151-5.

Chapter 11

RENAL BIOPSY WITH QUESTIONABLE INDICATIONS

INTRODUCTION

Insufficient international coordination of medical research and partial isolation from the international scientific community can result in repetition of studies performed in other countries. Renal biopsy (RB) is a valuable diagnostic tool; it was broadly used in the former Soviet Union (SU). RB were taken for research from patients with glomerulonephritis (Gn), pyelonephritis, amyloidosis, renovascular hypertension (from both kidneys in some studies) [1-6], essential hypertension [2], in certain studies with mild proteinuria and/or hematuria [7, 8], alcoholism [9-17], diabetes mellitus [18], rheumatoid arthritis [19], and from children with urinary tract anomalies including those combined with hydronephrosis or pyelonephritis [20-23]. RB in renovascular hypertension was discussed in [24, 25] and here in Chapter 7. The electron microscopy was infrequently used for diagnostics in the former SU. Nevertheless, about one third of the biopsy cylinder was embedded in epoxy resin. The semi-thin epoxy resin sections were made for research but were not used for diagnostics, the latter being performed mainly on the basis of paraffin sections and immunofluorescence.

Renal Biopsy Research in Pyelonephritis

In the studies [26, 27], excisional RB were sampled during kidney-preserving operations such as lithotomy from patients with chronic or acute (including purulent) pyelonephritis. In the international literature, pyelonephritis is not listed among conditions where RB is indicated, while acute inflammation, infection and hydronephrosis are generally considered to be contraindications [28-30]. In the study [31], RBs were collected from patients with chronic pyelonephritis and hydronephrosis, while conclusions were based on linear correlations between ultrastructural morphometric and clinical indices. However, statistical significance of the correlation coefficients in this and some similar studies was overstated. A comparison with the reference tables [32] demonstrated that many claimed P-values were too high for the given values of the correlation coefficient and the number of correlation pairs [31, 33-35]; more details are in [25] and in Chapter 7. In a more recent study, "cytomembranes of the interstitial tissue of renal medullary layer" were studied in core RB collected during lithotomies from patients with urolithiasis and secondary pyelonephritis [36]. Core RB were taken from patients with pyelonephritis also by other researchers [37]. Fine-needle RB in acute pyelonephritis was performed and recommended in the recent study [38].

Renal Biopsy Research in Alcoholism

Among patients with alcoholism, biopsies were taken from kidneys, pancreas, liver, lung, salivary glands, stomach and skin, repeatedly in some cases [12, 13, 17]. It was concluded on the basis of a series of RB studies that a generalized cytoskeleton abnormality with accumulation of filaments of intermediate type in macrophages, epithelial and other cells is typical for the cell damage by ethanol or the "alcoholic disease" [9, 12, 13]. It is known that Mallory bodies, seen in alcoholic hepatitis and some other liver conditions, contain filaments of intermediate type; however, generalizations as per [9, 12, 13] have never been confirmed by other researchers. In any case, the cytoskeleton can be studied in experiments or post mortem. Another example: RBs were collected from 40 patients with chronic alcoholism and nephritic symptoms, whereas "intracapillary proliferative glomerulonephritis" was diagnosed in all cases [15]. In a later study by the same researchers, the histopathological findings in 40 from 43 patients with alcoholism and nephritic symptoms were morphologically classified as membranoproliferative (mesangiocapillary) Gn; while in 29 from 31 patients with nephritic symptoms without alcoholism "fibroplastic" Gn was diagnosed [16]. The striking difference between the two groups is indicative of the data trimming. Other invasive procedures (celiacography, endoscopic cholangiopancreatography etc.) were applied in alcoholics without clear indications [17]; more details are in Chapter 10. In the author's opinion, repeated biopsies from different organs, doubtful morphological descriptions and interpretations, call in question the indications for RB at least in a part of the studied alcoholics.

RENAL BIOPSY AND GLOMERULONEPHRITIS

RB was performed without sufficient indications also in some cases of suspected Gn, which is less obvious because in the Russian-language literature RB has been generally regarded to be indicated in suspected Gn [39-41]. In the internationally used handbooks, RB in isolated proteinuria and/or microhematuria without abnormal urine sediment or signs of progressive renal disease is generally regarded to be not indicated [28, 42, 43]. Indications for RB are sometimes formulated more liberally [29]; but an obvious prerequisite must be a high quality of morphological examination. In the former SU, RB were sometimes collected from patients with "inactive nephritic" or latent clinical forms of Gn with proteinuria and/or hematuria [39, 44-47]. At the same time, the classification of Gn has been different from that used internationally [30, 43, 48], which interfered with the implementation of practical recommendations from the international literature. For example, Gn classification applied in the former SU did not consider IgA nephropathy as a separate entity [39, 49-51]. IgA-nephropathy was not mentioned even in the article from a leading institution dedicated to the "hematuric form" of Gn [52]. IgA-nephropathy was usually diagnosed on RB as mesangioproliferative Gn (MG) and treated with corticosteroids and/or cytotoxic drugs [39, 53-60]. In newer editions controversies can be found; for example, in the textbook [61], IgA nephropathy and Berger's disease are discussed separately and different treatments are recommended for them. IgA nephropathy as a separate entity was criticized as a "manifestation of a classificational crisis" [62]. New classifications of Gn were proposed [63]. It should be mentioned here that in the study [63] morphometric methods proposed earlier [64, 65] were used without due references.

In the "National Manual" [66], probably the most authoritative Russian-language edition in nephrology, IgA-nephropathy and MG are discussed in one chapter titled "Mesangioproliferative (IgA) glomerulonephritis" (from Russian): "The term IgA nephropathy is used to designate an entity, the morphological equivalent of which is mesangioproliferative glomerulonephritis" [66]. This is partly at variance with the accepted knowledge, according to which glomeruli in IgA nephropathy may be normal at light microscopy or may show segmental mesangial proliferation confined to some glomeruli (focal proliferative Gn), diffuse mesangial proliferation (such as in MG) or, rarely, crescentic Gn. Heeling of focal lesions can result in focal glomerulosclerosis [43, 67, 68].

Comparisons of percentages of glomerular diseases diagnosed by RB in Moscow and Rostock in Germany (Table 11.1) [51, 69] are suggestive of the overdiagnosis of Gn in the former. Old equipment, such as the sledge Reichert microtomes from the 1930s, was used in many institutions. The author of this book participated in research [24] using epoxy resin sections cut by an LKB pyramitome with glass knives; after that he found it difficult to examine diagnostic paraffin sections, less clearly visualizing basement membranes and mesangial matrix. The paraffin slides were relatively thick, the thickness being uneven. Occasionally overstained thick sections can make impression of a glomerular capillary wall thickening. This is apparently the reason why membranous Gn was diagnosed in Moscow more than twice as frequently as in Rostock (Table 11.1).

Table 11.1. Percentages of glomerular diseases diagnosed by RB in Moscow and Rostock (1978-1983) [51]

Condition	Moscow	Rostock
Diffuse Gn	81.7	59.3
MG	55.5	40.2
Membranous GN	9.2	4.1
Minor glomerular Abnormalities	7.1	20.8 30% 1990-1999 [69]

The diagnosis of MG was used broadly, encompassing 49-60.8% of all Gn cases diagnosed by RB [50, 70, 71]. Epoxy resin sections and silver impregnation were not used for the diagnostics, while electron microscopy was applied only occasionally in some institutions. By means of these methods, the collecting box of MG could have been partly sorted out, excluding from it some cases morphologically bordering on the norm i.e., isolated proteinuria and/or hematuria without renal or systemic disease, not requiring immunosuppressive therapy. In such cases, histologically are often detected only minor glomerular abnormalities: mild mesangial widening and hypercellularity, scarce deposits of immunoglobulins and complement [72]. In conditions of insufficient quality of histological specimens, without silver impregnation and electron microscopy, such changes were sometimes overestimated and Gn overdiagnosed. As mentioned above, RB were collected from patients with the "inactive nephritic" or latent clinical types of Gn i.e., minimal proteinuria and/or hematuria [39, 44-47]. As a result of the histological overdiagnosis of Gn, some of such patients were treated by corticosteroids and/or cytotoxic drugs such as azathioprin, cyclophosphamide or chlorambucil [53-60], without sufficient indications.

Renal Biopsy in Congenital Urinary Tract Abnormalities

The dubious concept of hypoplastic renal dysplasia was developed on the basis of pediatric RB. It was described as follows: "Racemosely arranged glomeruli with single capillary loops, abundant rounded cells freely lying in the cavity of a capsule; single mesangial cells; irregular enlargement, loosening, and thinning of the basement membrane", narrow extracapillary space, glomeruli having irregular form and singular capillary loops or total absence of capillaries [63, 73], which has no analogues in the international literature, where the terms "renal hypoplasia" and "dysplasia" are used with other meanings [74-77]. In the author's opinion, the descriptions were at least in part based on tangential sections of glomeruli, which is evident looking at the illustrations in [63, 73] partly reproduced in [78] (Figure 1.1). The authors were proposed to verify their concept counting glomeruli "with singular capillary loops" in autopsy or nephrectomy specimens, but it has not been done. Interestingly, one and the same ultrastructural image was published with a similar caption by different authors in the same journal 25 years apart [73, 79] (Figure 1.1). The common feature of these and some other works is the presentation of ultrastructural findings without confrontation with the light-microscopic picture, whereas variants of the norm and artefacts have been interpreted as specific pathological phenomena. For example, hypoplastic dysplasia was diagnosed by electron microscopy in 8 from 34 randomly selected patients aged 9-54 years with nephrotic syndrome and histologically minimal glomerular changes [80]. At the same time, there was no one case of Alport syndrome or thin basement membrane nephropathy (having some morphological features in common with the "hypoplastic dysplasia" as per [63, 73]) among 4440 RBs overviewed in [70]. These two conditions constituted ≥1% of all renal diseases diagnosed by RB in Rostock [69]. The concept of hypoplastic dysplasia, discussed with clinicians performing biopsies, could have interfered with the diagnosis of thin basement membrane nephropathy and Alport syndrome. The morphological diagnosis of both conditions is of importance for a genetic consultation of patients.

Today, the same researchers (or their heirs) apply the term hypoplastic dysplasia to the glomerular changes in congenital hydronephrosis and other renal abnormalities in children, interpreting them as an inborn nephropathy affecting a major part of glomeruli [20, 22, 79, 81, 82]. Note that a regular combination of two prima facie unrelated conditions: an inborn glomerulopathy affecting a major part of glomeruli, and hydronephrosis related to an abnormality of the ureteropelvic junction, seems to be improbable. Glomerular changes in hydronephrosis caused by the urine retention (collapse of the glomerular tuft with the widening of the urinary space) are different from those described according to the concept of hypoplastic dysplasia [79]. For this research, 167 intra-operative RBs from children with urogenital malformations, plus 18 RB for the control group from adult urological patients, were collected [82] with questionable indications at least in a part of the cases.

Renal and Pancreatic Biopsies in Diabetes Mellitus

The same group of researchers collected 60 pancreatic excision biopsies 5 × 5 mm in size [83] in the course of the surgical operations "pancreatic blood shunting into the systemic blood flow in insulin-dependent diabetics" [84] (discussed in Chapter 10). From the same patients, 51 core RBs were taken [83]. Apart from several reports from the former SU, we have found in the literature no analogues of this surgical treatment modality of diabetes mellitus [85] (More details are in Chapter 10). In the studies of RB from diabetics, Gn and mesangiolysis were designated as consecutive stages of diabetic glomerulosclerosis [86]. Ultrastructural descriptions included frequent mesangial interposition with displacement of mesangial cells to the periphery of glomerular capillary loops and formation of double-contour basement membranes [86, 87], which is at variance with usual descriptions [88-92]. In particular, the morphological picture of Gn, if detected in a diabetic patient, is usually interpreted as a superimposed condition possibly needing a special therapy [90, 91]. It should be commented that in diabetes mellitus, RB is generally indicated for patients under the suspicion of a renal disease other than diabetic nephropathy [93]. It is important to diagnose a non-diabetic renal condition, in particular, membranoproliferative Gn (characterized by the mesangial interposition), where the immunosuppressive therapy should be considered. Therefore, presenting the morphological picture of Gn as a characteristic phenomenon or a stage of diabetic nephropathy can be misleading.

CONCLUSION

The RB material used in some studies discussed above was unique e.g., wedge or core biopsies in hydronephrosis, acute and chronic pyelonephritis. Apart from the articles discussed here, no other studies based on RBs in hydronephrosis and acute pyelonephritis are known to us, while in chronic pyelonephritis no other studies performed abroad since the 1960s have been found. There is an opinion, shared by the author, that, considering potential complications, “RB for research” should not exist as such; it must always be performed according to clinical indications. If a patient gives informed consent to research on renal tissue obtained for diagnostic purposes, it can be done, provided that enough tissue remains for the diagnostics. Even today, the principle of informed consent is sometimes disregarded. At a reception of some governmental medical institutions a patient is given a form, where he or she must beforehand give a written consent to all diagnostic and therapeutic procedures, which are then sometimes performed in spite of the patient’s objections. In conclusion, high level of integrity, quality of specimens and of their examination must be a precondition for RB research. The problem is still with us: invasive procedures performed without sufficient clinical indications and informed consent.

REFERENCES

[1] Romanenko AM, Nosov AT, Pereverzev AS, Zubko VI. Morphologic changes of the kidneys in patients with vasorenal hypertension. *Vrach Delo* 1989;(6):35-8.

[2] Shkhvatsabaia IK, Iurenev AP, Kozdoba OA. Lesions of target organs in arterial hypertension. *Kardiologiia* 1986;26(10):75-80.

[3] Pal'tsev MA, Iargin SV, Krotovskii GS, Turpitko SA, Mamedov DM. Importance of morphologic examination of the kidneys of patients with vasorenal hypertension for predicting the results of surgical treatment. *Arkh Patol* 1986;48(6):34-40.

[4] Pal'tsev MA, Krotovski GS, Egorova IA, Shcherbiuk AN. State of the neuroendocrine aparatus of the kidney during renovascular hypertension as a criterion of the prognosis of the surgery outcome. *Arkh Patol* 1982;44(8):62-71.

[5] Turpitko SA, Iargin SV, Petrovskii PF, Klembovskii AA, Gerasimov VB. Angiographic and morphologic criteria of the manifestation of arteriolonephrosclerosis in vasorenal hypertension. *Urol Nefrol* (Mosk) 1989;(2):34-37.

[6] Pal'tsev MA, Iargin SV, Krotovskii GS, Turpitko SA, Kazanchan PO. Relation of the effectiveness of surgical treatment of vasorenal hypertension and morphologic changes of the kidneys. *Kardiologiia* 1989;29(4):76-80.

[7] Arabidze GG, Sokolova RI, Titov VN, Tarasov AV. The diagnosis of hypertension (research on kidney biopsies and microalbuminuria. *Ter Arkh* 1989;61(9):8-12.

[8] Nichik TE, Kayukov IG, Essaian AM. Morphological alterations to the kidneys in arterial hypertension combined with mild proteinuria. *Nefrologiia* 2006;10(4):66-71.

[9] Serov VV, Lebedev SP. Clinical morphology of alcoholism. *Arkh Patol 1985*;47(8):3-14.

[10] Nikolaev Alu, Serov VV, Tareeva IE, Varshavskii VA, Lebedev SP. Clinicomorphological characteristics and prognosis of glomerulonephritis in chronic alcoholism. *Ter Arkh 1986*;58(8):115-20.

[11] Lebedev SP, Kovtun TI, Sukhova GK. Morphology and various problems of the pathogenesis of alcoholic microangiopathy. *Arkh Patol* 1986;48(10):26-33.

[12] Lebedev SP, Vinogradova LG, Sukhova GK. Alcoholic hyaline and interstitial filaments as markers of alcoholic damage of internal organs. *Arkh Patol* 1984;46(11):52-58.

[13] Serov VV, Lebedev SP. *Clinical morphology of visceral alcoholism.* Vestn Akad Med Nauk SSSR 1988;(3):48-53.

[14] Serov VV, Lebedev SP, Vinogradova LG, Mukhin AS, Sukhova GK. Intermediate filaments in the lung macrophages and endothelial cells in chronic alcoholism and supurativedestructive lung diseases. *Biull Eksp Biol Med* 1982;94(12):92-94.

[15] Tarasova NS, Beloborodova EI. Immunological aspects of circulating immune complexes in kidney diseases in patients with chronic alcoholism. *Ter Arkh* 1998;70(12):61-63.

[16] Tarasova NS, Beloborodova EI. Hormonal and immunological aspects of renal lesions in patients with chronic alcoholism. *Ter Arkh* 2003;75(11):73-76.

[17] Makhov VM, Abdullin RG, Gitel' EL, Zavodnov VIa, Podzolkov VI, et al. Visceral lesions in alcoholism. Ter Arkh 1996;68(8):53-56.

[18] Mukhin NA, Dedov II, Shestakova MV, Pal'tsev MA, Varshavskii VA, et al. The functional kidney reserves of diabetics. *Ter Arkh* 1990;62(2):107-10.

[19] Khamishon LZ, Chichasova NB, Kanevskaia MZ, Varshavskii VA, Semeikina OV, et al. Glomerulonephritis in rheumatoid arthritis. *Revmatologiia* 1989;(4):18-23.

[20] Severgina LO, Leonova LV, Severgina ES, Gurevich AI, Menovshchikova LB, et al. Coupling between the hemodynamic parameters and the morphological changes in the kidney in children with congenital hydronephrosis. *Arkh Patol* 2011;73(2):14-17.

[21] Kozhukhova OA, Klembovski AI. Morphological manifestations of disorders of renal tissue differentiation in children. *Arkh Patol* 1979;41(10):6-13.

[22] Leonova LV, Severgina ES, Popova OP, Konovalov DM, Petruchina IuV, et al. Transforming growth factor as a marker beta of nephrogenetic disturbance in congenital obstructive uropathies. *Arkh Patol* 2007;69(4):35-38.

[23] Cheskis AL, Leonova LV, Severgina ES, Ostapko MS, Simonova NA, et al. Renal development long after correction of primary nonrefluxing forms of megaureter in children. *Urologiia* 2006;(5):74-80.

[24] Jargin SV. Some Aspects of Renal Biopsy for Research. Int J Nephrol Kidney Failure 20151(2): doi: 10.16966/2380-5498.108.

[25] Jargin SV. *Manipulation with statistics in medical research.* Dermatopathology: Practical & Conceptual 2009;15:21.

[26] Kirillov IuA. Morphogenesis of acute pyelonephritis (electron microscopic study). *Arkh Patol* 1979;41(8):29-36.

[27] Kirillov IuA. Morphogenesis of chronic pyelonephritis (electron microscopic study). *Arkh Patol* 1980;42(1):38-45.

[28] Kasiske BL, Keane WF. Laboratory assessment of renal disease: clearance, urinalysis, and renal biopsy. In: Brenner BM (ed) Brenner & Rector's *The Kidney.* 6th edition. Philadelphia: W.B. Saunders, 2000; 129-70.

[29] Tomson CR. Indications for renal biopsy in chronic kidney disease. *Clin Med* 2003;3:513-7.

[30] Tischer CC, Wilcox CS. *Nephrology.* 3rd edition, Baltimore: Williams & Wilkins, 1995.

[31] Pal'tsev MA. Juxtaglomerular aparatus and interstitial cells of kidney medulla in hydronephrosis and chronic pyelonephritis. *Arkh Patol* 1982;44(5):12-19.

[32] Lentner C. *Wissenschaftliche Tabellen Geigi* [Scientific tables Geigi]. Basel: CIBA-GEIGI, 1980.

[33] Serov VV, Pal'tsev MA. Endocrine system of the kidneys in nephrogenic arterial hypertension: functional and morphological analysis. *Arkh Patol* 1984;46(11):5-16.

[34] Pal'tsev MA, Bespalov DA, Shliapnikov VV, Kutyrina IM, Nikishova TA. Juxtaglomerular aparatus and interstitial cells of the kidney medulla in glomerulonephritis. *Arkh Patol* 1984;46(2):64-70.

[35] Mukhin NA, Popova EN, Fomin VV, Popova IA, Kuznetsova AV, et al. Clinical significance of markers of endothelial dysfunction and angiogenesis in progressing of the lung interstitial diseases. *Ross Fiziol Zh Im I M Sechenova* 2009;95(10):1139-50.

[36] Kazeko NI, Zhmurov VA, Borovskii AA, Veshkurtsev VV, Khvan OV. Lipids content in renal tissue membranes in patients with urolithiasis and secondary pyelonephritis. *Urologiia* 2005;(5):56-58.

[37] Shulutko BI, Kulaeva NN, Ambrozas IV, Shumilkin VR, Anikonova LI. The clinical significance of immunological indices in chronic pyelonephritis. *Ter Arkh* 1993;65(6):11-13.

[38] Diusiubaev AA, Shalashov VA. Thin needle aspiration biopsy of the kidneys in diagnosis of acute pyelonephritis. *Urologiia* 2007;(6): 29-31.

[39] Shilov EM, Tareeva IE, Ivanov AA, Troepol'skaia OV, Krasnova TN, et al. The course and prognosis of mesangioproliferative glomerulonephritis. *Ter Arkh* 2002;74(6):11-18.

[40] Borisov VV, Vashurina TV, Voznesenskaya TS. Clinical recommendations according to syndromes. In: Mukhin NA, Fomin VV (eds) *Nephrology. National Manual.* Moscow: Geotar-media, 2009; 93-161. (Russian)

[41] Lozinskii EIu. *Clinical nephrology.* Vladivostok: Far Eastern Federal Univ., 2007. (Russian)

[42] Tisher CC. Clinical indications for kidney biopsy. In: Tisher CC, Brenner BM (eds) *Renal pathology*. Philadelphia: Lipincott, 1989; pp. 2-10.

[43] Black RM. *Rose & Black's clinical problems in nephrology*. Boston: Little, Brown and Co., 1996.

[44] Ratner MIa, Fedorova ND, Makurov AI. The tubulointerstitial changes in different clinical and morphological types of chronic glomerulonephritis. *Urol Nefrol* (Mosk) 1997;(2):16-19.

[45] Varshavskii VA, Laurinavichius AA, Zhigalin VG. Characteristics of primary glomerulonephritis (on the basis of kidney biopsies of the Pathology Department, I.M. Sechenov Moscow Medical Academy, from 1980 to 1989). *Arkh Patol* 1992;54(6):36-40.

[46] Ratner M, Serov VV, Warschavski WA, Rosenfeld B, Subkin ML, et al. Recommendations for a clinical classification of chronic glomerulonephritis. *Z Urol Nephrol* 1987;80:271-9.

[47] Chebotareva NV, Neprintseva NV, Bobkova IN, Kozlovskaia LV.. Investigation of 70-kDa heat shock protein in the serum and urine of patients with chronic glomerulonephritis. *Ter Arkh* 2014;86(6): 18-23.

[48] Churg J, Bernstein J, Glassock RJ. *Renal disease: Classification and atlas of glomerular diseases.* 2nd edition. New York: Igaku-Shoin, 1995.

[49] Serov VV. The purpose of clinical morphology is diagnosis. *Klin Med* (Mosk) 1990;68(4):143-144.

[50] Ratner MIa, Serov VV, Rozenfel'd BI, Varshavskii VA, Brodskii MA. Clinico-morphological variants and prognosis of chronic glomerulonephritis. *Ter Arkh* 1983;55(6):10-14.

[51] Serov VV, Varshavsky VA, Schill H, Nizze H. Incidence of glomerular diseases in kidney biopsy materials using WHO classification. *Zentralbl Allg Pathol* 1986;132:471-5.

[52] Ratner MIa, Serov VV, Varshavskii VA, Brodskii MA, Makurov AI. Functional and morphological characteristics of a hematuric form of chronic glomerulonephritis. *Klin Med* (Mosk) 1990;68(6):54-57.

[53] Ratner MIa, Tomilina NA, Klinkman Kh, Shmitt E, Kreger E. Prolonged treatment of mesangioproliferative glomerulonephritis with a cytostatic agent and prednisolone and a combination of a cytostatic agent, prednisolone an anticoagulant and an antiaggregant. *Ter Arkh* 1980;52(8):106-10.

[54] Ratner MIa, Biriukova LS, Makurov AI. Indications and effectiveness of combined therapy in chronic glomerulonephritis. *Ter Arkh* 1987;59(8):29-34.

[55] Ratner MIa, Serov VV, Stenina IN, Fedorova ND, Shumakov VI. The importance of the clinical classification of chronic glomerulonephritis for the prognosis of its progression and of the efficacy of therapy. *Ter Arkh* 1996;68(6):10-13.

[56] Tareeva IE, Gordovskaia NB, Gladskikh OP, Ivanov AA, Krasnova TN. Treatment of chronic glomerulonephritis with cytostatics. *Ter Arkh* 1989;61(6):9-14.

[57] Ratner MIa, Tomilina NA, Serov VV. Long-term use of a combination of immunosupressants, and antiaggregant and an anticoagulant in the treatment of glomerulonephritis. *Ter Arkh* 1979;51(6):43-47.

[58] Serov VV, Pal'tsev MA, Mukhin NA, Tareeva IE, Kozlovskaia (Lysenko) LV, et al. The key problems of glomerulonephritis. *Ter Arkh* 1992;64(6):5-10.

[59] Krasnova TN, Shilov EM, Ivanov AA, Samoilov DV, Gordovskaia NB, et al. The treatment of chronic glomerulonephritis with ultrahigh doses of cyclophosphane. *Ter Arkh* 1991;63(6):115-8.

[60] Poliantseva LR, Gordovskaia NB, Krasnova TN, Samoilov DV, Shilov EM. Complications induced by cytostatic therapy of glomerulonephritis. *Ter Arkh* 1990;62(12):63-66.

[61] Stepanov OG. Nephrology. *Textbook for postgraduate students.* Maikop: Kucherenko, 2013. (in Russian)

[62] Pyrig LA, Mel'man NIa, Romanenko AM. Principles of clinical morphology in nephrology. *Klin Med* (Mosk) 1989;67(4):152-4.

[63] Varshavskii VA, Proskurneva EP, Gasanov AB, Severgina LO, Shestakova LA. Subdivision of certain morphological variants of chronic glomerulonephritis. *Arkh Patol* 1999;61(5):40-46.

[64] Jargin SV. Morphological characteristics of nephrosclerosis of different etiologies. *Arkh Patol* 1985;47(10):62-70.

[65] Iargin SV. Nosological characteristics of the morphogenesis of nephrosclerosis. *Arkh Patol* 1986;48(7):55-63.

[66] Shilov EM. Mesangioproliferative (IgA) glomerulonephritis. In: Mukhin NA, Fomin VV (eds) *Nephrology. National manual.* Short edition. Moscow: Geotar-media, 2014; pp. 214-22. (in Russian)

[67] Schrier RW. *Manual of nephrology.* 5th edition. Philadelphia: Lipincott Williams & Wilkins, 2000.

[68] Cotran RS, Kumar V, Robbins SL. *Robbins' Pathologic Basis of Disease.* 5th edition. Philadelphia: Saunders, 1994.

[69] Nizze H, Mann E, Stropahl G, Schmidt W. Glomerular diseases in renal biopsy. Correlation of clinical syndromes with histological types. *Pathologe* 2003;24:421-32.

[70] Dzhanaliev BR, Varshavskii VA, Laurinavicius AA. Primary glomerulopathies: incidence, dynamics and clinical manifestations of morphological variants. *Arkh Patol* 2002;64(2):32-35.

[71] Ratner MIa, Serov VV, Varshavskii VA, Novikov ID, Rozenfel'd BI. New classification of chronic glomerulonephritis. *Klin Med* (Mosk) 1987;65(4):6-11.

[72] Churg J, Sobin LH. *Renal disease. Classification and atlas of glomerular diseases.* Tokyo: Igaku-Shoin, 1982.

[73] Severgina ES, Pal'tsev MA. Hypoplastic dysplasia as one of the forms of nephropathy. *Arkh Patol* 1989;51(10):58-63.

[74] Squiers EC, Morden RS, Bernstein J. Renal multicystic dysplasia: an occasional manifestation of the hereditary renal adysplasia syndrome. In: Opitz JM, Bernstein J, Spano LM (eds) *Topics in pediatric genetic pathology.* New York: Wiley-Liss, 1987; pp. 279-84.

[75] Kakkar N, Menon S, Radotra BD. Histomorphology of renal dysplasia - an autopsy study. *Fetal Pediatr Pathol* 200;625:73-86.

[76] Woolf AS, Price KL, Scambler PJ, Winyard PJ. Evolving concepts in human renal dysplasia. *J Am Soc Nephrol* 2004;15: 998-1007.

[77] Botvin'ev OK, Safinova MP. Clinical and morphological characteristics of renal hypoplasia in children. *Arkh Patol* 2014; 76(1):42-44.

[78] Jargin SV. Pancreatic and renal biopsy for research: back to the indications. *Molodoi Uchenyi Young Sci* 2014;(4):143-7.

[79] Severgina LO, Gurevich SI. Ultrastructural assessment of the role of dysangiogenesis in congenital hydronephrosis. *Arkh Patol* 2014;76(6):51-55.

[80] Severgina ES. Ultrastructural heterogeneity of "minimal changes" in the kidney glomeruli, detected by light optics. *Arkh Patol* 1991;53(2):53-8.

[81] Cheskis AL, Severgina ES, Leonova LV, Ostapko MS. Status and development of the kidney after surgical treatment of hydronephrosis in children. *Urologiia* 2002;(4):39-43.

[82] Severgina LO. *The role of dysangiogenesis in malformations of the urogenital system.* Higher doctorate thesis. Moscow: I.M. Sechenov Medical Academy, 2014.

[83] Severgina ES. *Morphology and pathogenesis of insulindependent diabetes mellitus.* Higher doctorate thesis. Moscow: I.M. Sechenov Medical Academy, 1995.

[84] Galperin EI, Diuzheva TG, Petrovsky PF, Chevokin AYu, Dokuchayev KV, et al. Results of pancreatic blood shunting into the systemic blood flow in insulin-dependent diabetics. *HPB Surg* 1996;9:191-7.

[85] Jargin SV. Surgical procedures with questionable indications: a letter from Russia. J Surgery 2016;4(1):6.

[86] Severgina ES, Ponomarev AB, Diuzheva TG, Shestakova MV, Maiorova EM. Diabetic glomerulonephritis - the first stage of diabetic glomerulopathy. *Arkh Patol* 1994;56(4):44-50.

[87] Severgina ES, Ponomarev AB, Diuzheva TG, Shestakova MV, Maiorova EM. Diabetic glomerulosclerosis - a prolonged stage of diabetic glomerulopathy. *Arkh Patol* 1994;56(4):50-55.

[88] Spencer J, Peakman M. Post-mortem analysis of islet pathology in type 1 diabetes illuminates the life and death of the beta cell. *Clin Exp Immunol* 2009;155:125-7.

[89] Richardson SJ, Morgan NG, Foulis AK. Pancreatic Pathology in Type 1 Diabetes Mellitus. *Endocr Pathol 2014*;25:80-92.

[90] Dizdar O, Kahraman S, Gençtoy G, Ertoy D, Arici M, et al. Membranoproliferative glomerulonephritis associated with type 1 diabetes mellitus and Hashimoto's thyroiditis. *Nephrol Dial Transplant* 2004;19:988-9.

[91] Hironaka K, Makino H, Ikeda S, Haramoto T, Ota Z. Nondiabetic renal disease complicating diabetic nephropathy. *J Diabet Complications* 1991;5:148-9.

[92] Hanafusa T, Miyazaki A, Miyagawa J, Tamura S, Inada M, et al. Examination of islets in the pancreas biopsy specimens from newly diagnosed type 1 (insulin-dependent) diabetic patients. *Diabetologia* 1990;33:105-11.

[93] Gonzalez Suarez ML, Thomas DB, Barisoni L, Fornoni A. Diabetic nephropathy: Is it time yet for routine kidney biopsy? *World J Diabetes* 2013;4:245-55.

Chapter 12

Consequences of the Chernobyl Accident

On the basis of the linear no-threshold theory (LNT), Chernobyl accident was predicted to result in a considerable increase in radiation-induced cancer. In fact, there has been no cancer incidence increase proven to be a consequence of the radiation exposure except for thyroid cancer (TC) in people exposed at a young age [1]. The reliability of early reports of a TC increase after the accident was doubted as radioiodine was thought to have low carcinogenicity [2]. High incidence and the short latent period were deemed unusual; the number of TC in children and adolescents exposed to radiation has been higher than expected on the basis of previous knowledge [1, 3]. There was uncertainty about the accuracy of diagnoses [4].

The Chernobyl accident gives an example of considerable difference in diagnostic quality before and after the event. Introduction of the ultrasonography and fine needle aspiration biopsy (FNAB), coupled with a superficial location of the thyroid gland, resulted in the detection of large numbers of thyroid nodules, while "radiation phobia" [5], suboptimal quality of histological specimens and insufficient experience with pediatric material contributed to the overdiagnosis of malignancy. Availability of children at schools and preschools for the mass screening explains for the

TC incidence increase predominantly in this age group [6]. The registered incidence of pediatric TC in the former Soviet Union (SU) before the accident was low compared to other developed nations, which had obviously been caused by differences in diagnostic quality and coverage of the population by medical examinations [7]. Accordingly, there was a pool of undiagnosed TC prior to the accident. The percentage of more advanced (deemed aggressive radiogenic) cancers was negatively associated with the time between the accident and surgery [8-10] probably due to the gradual exhaustion by the screening of the pool of advanced cancers.

There were several factors predisposing the over-diagnosis of TC. Equipment of histopathological laboratories was outdated in the 1990s; excessive thickness of histological sections hindered reliable assessment of morphological criteria. Gross dissection of surgical specimens was often made with blunt knives, without rinsing instruments and the board for cutting, often without access to water [11], which can result in the tissue deformation and contamination of the cut surface by cells mimicking malignancy criteria. It can explain for the high frequency of "ingrowths of tumor cells into blood vessels" found in post-Chernobyl pediatric TC in 45% of cases [12]. Pathologists in Russia, who worked with thyroid tumors from contaminated areas, pointed out the low quality of histological specimens interfering with evaluation of nuclei [13].

False-positive diagnosis of TC was not excluded after cytological and histological examinations. One of the mechanisms has been as follows. If a thyroid nodule is found by an ultrasonic screening, FNAB is normally performed. Thyroid FNAB cytology has a certain percentage of inconclusive results [14], which must have been relatively high in the former SU, one of the causes being shortage of modern literature [15]. The data about sensitivity of the FNAB in detecting of post-Chernobyl childhood TC were reported: "In a definite or presumptive form, diagnosis of carcinoma was established in 161 from 238 cases", while papillary carcinoma was diagnosed correctly by FNA in 69.5% and follicular subtype of papillary TC - only in 36.5% of cases [16]. After receiving a cytological report in a presumptive form (suspicious for malignancy), a hemithyroidectomy, subtotal or total thyroidectomy has been performed

[12, 17]. After 1991, the total thyroidectomy predominated [12]. The prevalent opinion was that surgical treatment of radiogenic TC must be "more radical" than usual, while subtotal thyroidectomy was regarded "oncologically not justified" [18]. The surgical specimen is sent for pathological examination. After the in toto removal of a supposed cancer, a pathologist may confirm malignancy also in cases with equivocal histology. The data about verification by expert commissions of post-Chernobyl pediatric TC in Russia confirmed the fact of false-positivity: "As a result of histopathological verification, diagnosis of TC was confirmed in 79.1% of cases (federal level of verification - 354 cases) and 77.9% (international level - 280 cases)" [16]. False-positive cases, not covered by verifications, have remained undisclosed, the more so as archives of histological specimens were in disarray also in some central institutions, slides often "taken by relatives for external consultations" etc. thus becoming unavailable for checkups. Some diagnostic criteria of TC were not mentioned by Russian-language literature used at that time [19, 20]. One of the most important diagnostic criteria of papillary TC - the ground-glass or cleared nuclei - was mistranslated as "watch-glass nuclei" and presented by the most authoritative Russian-language handbook of tumor pathology [20] as a feature not only of papillary, but also of follicular TC. Nuclear features, typical for papillary carcinoma, are not visible in the illustrations of this handbook [20]. In the widely used Atlas of tumor histopathology [21], the following is stated about thyroid nodules: "In severe dysplasia there appear cell groups with clearly visible atypia. Therefore, the 3rd grade dysplasia is considered as an obligate pre-cancer, which histologically is hardly distinguishable from carcinoma in situ" [21]. Accordingly, the diagnostic formulations such as "follicular thyroid carcinoma without invasion" or "follicular carcinoma in situ", suggestive of false-positivity, could be encountered [16]. Note that nuclear atypia is generally not regarded as a malignancy criterion of thyroid nodules; and the concepts of carcinoma in situ and dysplasia are not applied to them [22]. Several images from [20, 21], potentially misleading for the practice, have been reproduced in [23, 24]. Cases of false-positive diagnosis, caused by a misinterpretation of nuclear atypia as a malignancy criterion of

thyroid nodules, are known from practice. The articles describing mechanisms of the false-positivity, possibly active until today, have been rejected by the main journal of Russian pathologists Arkhiv Patologii (Archives of Pathology) despite repeated personal communications with the Editor-in-Chief Georgii Frank and co-editor Irina Voloshchuk. As a result, the articles about the false-positivity and overtreatment of Chernobyl-related lesions have been published abroad and in Russian journals that are usually not read by pathologists [6, 7, 25].

After the Chernobyl accident, numerous poorly substantiated publications appeared, where spontaneous diseases in Chernobyl clean-up workers and inhabitants of radiocontaminated areas, sometimes quite distant from Chernobyl, were a priori considered to be radiogenic [26-31]. Previously we discussed several publications overestimating medical consequences of Chernobyl accident [6, 7, 25]. Unreliability of others can be inferred by analogy: if earlier papers on the same topic were unreliable, later ones might be unreliable as well, because motivations and the attitude remained unchanged. For an inside observer it is evident that behind the avalanche of Russian-language papers, overestimating Chernobyl consequences (some of them referenced in [31]) was a directive, which was not unusual for the Soviet science. Research topics were often assigned to the scientists, while "expected results" were discussed at Scientific Councils (uchenyi soviet) sometimes being, in fact, suggested in advance. Desired research results could be "recommended" by a superior, which was favored by the authoritative management style, ingrained also in science and medicine. Motives for the overestimation of Chernobyl consequences have been obvious: it facilitated writing of dissertations, financing, international help, etc. The Chernobyl accident has been exploited to strangle worldwide development of atomic energy [32].

Travelling to the areas, formerly contaminated due to the Chernobyl accident, the author of this book interviewed pathologists, cytologists and other specialists, who participated in diagnostics of the post-Chernobyl tumors. Most of them agreed that Chernobyl consequences had been overestimated. It was also stated that sets of histological specimens from a single patient were sometimes subdivided into several ones, creating "dead souls", which influenced statistics. Radio- and cancerophobia, sometimes amounting to panic, contributed to the overdiagnosis of cancer, which can be illustrated by the following citations from a Russian-language professional publication (verbatim translation): "Practically all nodular thyroid lesions, independently of their size, were regarded at that time in children as potentially malignant tumors, requiring an urgent surgical operation" or "Aggressiveness of surgeons contributed to the shortening of the minimal latency period" [4]. Obviously, the mass screening in the areas, where pediatric TC had been rarely diagnosed before, on the background of poor equipment and shortage of modern literature, in the atmosphere of radio- and cancerophobia, of vested interests both in decision-making spheres and among researchers, must have inevitably resulted in overestimation. The principal causes of the overestimation of Chernobyl consequences likely include unreliability of Chernobyl-related (and some other) research, originating from the former SU, a nonchalant attitude towards scientific misconduct in general and manipulations with statistics in particular.

The misclassification of neglected advanced cases as aggressive radiogenic cancers gave rise to the concept that supposedly radiogenic thyroid cancers, at least those from the "first wave" after the accident, were more aggressive than sporadic ones [3, 8, 10, 33, 34]. This had consequences for the practice: the surgical treatment of supposedly radiogenic thyroid cancers was recommended to be "more radical" [18]. After 1998-1999, the surgery in some institutions of the former SU switched to a more aggressive approach [33, 35]. The following treatment was recommended to the children with radiogenic TC: "Total thyroidectomy combined with neck dissections followed by radioiodine ablation" [36]; "Careful and complete removal of the lymph nodes is of great clinical relevance" [37]. External radiotherapy (40 Gy) was applied as well [38]. The total thyroidectomy has been seen by some experts to be indicated regardless of the tumor size and histopathology [35, 36]; whereas technical difficulties of parathyroid glands preservation were pointed out [12]. Some experts regarded subtotal thyroidectomy to be oncologically not justified and advocated total thyroidectomy with a prophylactic neck dissection. Lesser resections were regarded to be "only acceptable in exceptional cases of very small solitary intrathyroidal carcinomas without evidence of neck lymph node involvement on surgical revision" [35]. It was written in a recent instructive publication that bilateral neck dissection must be performed in all cases independently of the tumor size, histology and lymph node status [39]. This is at variance with a more conservative treatment of thyroid carcinoma applied worldwide also in the settings of the Fukushima Daiichi nuclear accident [40]. The articles [41, 42] were misquoted by Demidchik and Kontratovich [43] advocating total thyroidectomy with bilateral neck dissection for all cases of pediatric thyroid cancer. Moreover, the sources [42, 44, 45] were cited in support of the statement: "The most prevailing opinion calls for total thyroidectomy regardless of tumor size and histopathology" [35]. In fact, the subtotal thyroidectomy was used or recommended in these articles, in some of them along with the total thyroidectomy [42, 44, 45]. Note that total thyroidectomy with neck dissection is associated with complications such as hypoparathyroidism and recurrent laryngeal nerve palsy [4, 17, 46, 47]. The high suicide rate noticed among patients with Chernobyl-related thyroid cancer [48, 49] can be explained by a decreased quality of life after the excessively radical surgery. Moreover, a majority of post-Chernobyl thyroid patients were young females potentially concerned about cosmetic aspects.

Remarkable data were reported about thyroid adenoma. The RET rearrangements were found in 57.1% of the adenomas in patients from non-contaminated areas of Ukraine but in 0% of thyroid adenomas from France [50]. This discrepancy was explained in the same article: at a re-examination, in 8 from 14 adenomas from Ukraine, but in no one from France, were found groups of cells with "limited nuclear features of papillary cancers" [50], which is indicative of uncertainty of the histopathological diagnostics. The diagnostic uncertainty is a possible explanation for the fact that in different groups of males with benign prostatic hyperplasia (BPH) and females with chronic cystitis, from contaminated areas and Kiev, severe urothelial dysplasia and carcinoma in situ (CIS) were found by the bladder biopsy as frequently as in 56-92% of all randomly selected cases; while the random selection mode was repeatedly pointed out [51-55]. Such a high prevalence of severe dysplasia and CIS in randomly selected BPH cases is unrealistic and indicative of false-positivity. Radiation doses resulting from activity concentration of ^{137}Cs in urine (6.47 Bq/l in the most exposed group [52, 53]) were discussed previously [56]: the doses were too low to cause any increase in the bladder malignancy. It should be stressed that the overdiagnosis of premalignant and malignant bladder lesions entails overtreatment and over-manipulation including cystoscopies and repeated biopsies [51-55], potentially conductive to a transmission of infection such as viral hepatitis. It seems to be probable that the so-called "irradiation cystitis" [53, 57], characterized not only by urothelial dysplasia and CIS but also by "reactive epithelial proliferation associated with hemorrhage, fibrin deposits, fibrinoid vascular changes, and multinuclear stromal cells" [57] was at least in part caused or maintained by repeated cystoscopies, mapping biopsies, electrocoagulation etc. It can be reasonably assumed that some of molecular markers, especially those associated with tissue damage, inflammation and cell proliferation (TGF-β1, p38 mitogen-activated protein kinases, growth factors, etc.), as well as the "marked activation of angiogenesis in urinary bladder lamina propria" [53], reflected chronic inflammation and increased cellular proliferation unrelated to ionizing radiation and possibly iatrogenic. In this regard, the images from [53, 55], reproduced in [24, 58, 59] should be commented. All the slides were evidently too thick for reliable diagnostics, nuclei are weakly stained. Insufficient quality of specimens could have been caused also by fixation- and processing-related factors, tissue damage due to electrocoagulation etc. Some images from [53, 55], published 9 years apart, were identical. Histological images of bladder and thyroid lesions, potentially conductive to false-positive diagnosis, can be seen in broadly used editions on tumor histopathology [20, 21, 60], some of them reproduced and commented in [6, 23, 58, 61].

Conclusion

Medical consequences of the Chernobyl accident have been overestimated in many publications. Advanced neglected cancers found during the first decade after the Chernobyl accident by the screening, or brought from non-contaminated areas and registered as Chernobyl victims, were misinterpreted as rapidly growing radiogenic malignancies [6, 7, 61]. Various kinds of bias can be found in the epidemiological research reporting increased cancer risks from low-dose radiation: classification of spontaneous diseases as radiation-induced, analyses of doses disregarding natural radiation background, conclusions about incidence increase without adequate control, "forcing a positive slope to the relative risk dose-response curve" [62] i.e., data trimming, as well as misquoting and tendentious citation [63, 64]. The misquoting was used for the purpose of exaggeration of Chernobyl consequences e.g., by Mikhail Balonov [64]. Other bias and confounders have been discussed [25, 65, 66]. The enhanced attention to the topic facilitated international cooperation, financing and foreign aid. Numerous papers and dissertations have been written for scientific careers, some of them being of questionable reliability [25, 63]. The above and previously published [6, 7, 12, 61] arguments call into question the validity of cause-effect relationships between radiation exposures after the accident and the cancer incidence increase. With regard to TC in people exposed as children and adolescents, such relationship is not excluded. However, the number of radiogenic cancers has been overestimated, which may lead to a wrong carcinogenicity concept of low-dose low-rate exposures, especially from radioiodine.

References

[1] UNSCEAR 2000 Report to the General Assembly. Annex J. *Exposures and effects of the Chernobyl accident*. New York: United Nations, 2000.

[2] Williams D. Thyroid growth and cancer. *Eur Thyroid J* 2015;4:164-73.

[3] IARC. Thyroid cancer in young people. In: Ionizing radiation, part 2: some internally deposited radionuclides. Views and expert opinions of an IARC Working Group on the Evaluation of Carcinogenic Risks to Humans. Lyon, 14-21 June 2000. *IARC Monogr Eval Carcinog Risks Hum* 2001;78(Pt 2):233-236.

[4] Lushnikov EF, Tsyb AF, Yamashita S. *Thyroid cancer in Russia after the Chernobyl.* Moscow: Meditsina, 2006.

[5] Mould RF. *Chernobyl record. The definite history of the Chernobyl catastrophe*. Philadelphia: Institute of Physics, 2000.

[6] Jargin SV. Some aspects of thyroid neoplasia after Chernobyl. *Hamdan Med J* 2020;13:69-77.

[7] Jargin SV. Chernobyl-Related Cancer and Precancerous Lesions: Incidence Increase vs. Late Diagnostics. *Dose Response* 2014;12:404-14.

[8] Williams ED, Abrosimov A, Bogdanova T, Demidchik EP, Ito M, et al. Thyroid carcinoma after Chernobyl latent period, morphology and aggressiveness. *Br J Cancer* 2004;90:2219-24.

[9] Bogdanova TI, Zurnadzhy LY, Nikiforov YE, Leeman-Neill RJ, Tronko MD, et al. Histopathological features of papillary thyroid carcinomas detected during four screening examinations of a Ukrainian-American cohort. *Br J Cancer* 2015;113:1556-64.

[10] Zablotska LB, Nadyrov EA, Rozhko AV, Gong Z, Polyanskaya ON, et al. Analysis of thyroid malignant pathologic findings identified during 3 rounds of screening (1997-2008) of a cohort of children and adolescents from Belarus exposed to radioiodines after the Chernobyl accident. *Cancer* 2015;121:457-66.

[11] Jargin SV. The practice of pathology in Russia: On the eve of modernization. *Basic Appl Pathol* 2010;3:70-73.

[12] Demidchik EP, Tsyb AF, Lushnikov EF. Thyroid carcinoma in children. *Consequences of Chernobyl accident* (in Russian). Meditsina, Moscow, 1996.

[13] Abrosimov AIu, Lushnikov EF, Frank GA. Radiogenic (Chernobyl) thyroid cancer. *Arkh Patol* 2001;63(4):3-9.

[14] Le AR, Hompson GW, Hoyt BJ. Thyroid fine-needle aspiration biopsy: an evaluation of its utility in a community setting. *J Otolaryngol Head Neck Surg* 2015;44:12.

[15] Murphy J, Jargin S. International trends in health science librarianship part 20: Russia. *Health Info Libr J* 2017;34(1):92-94.

[16] Abrosimov AIu. *Thyroid carcinoma in children and adolescents of Russian Federation after the Chernobyl accident.* Doctoral dissertation. Obninsk: Medical Radiological Research Centre, 2004.

[17] Rybakov SJ, Komissarenko IV, Tronko ND, Kvachenyuk AN, Bogdanova TI, et al. Thyroid cancer in children of Ukraine after the Chernobyl accident. *World J Surg* 2000;24:1446-9.

[18] Rumiantsev PO. *Thyroid cancer: modern approaches to diagnostics and treatment.* Moscow: Geotar-Media, 2009.

[19] Bomash NIu. *Morphological diagnostics of thyroid diseases.* Moscow: Meditsina, 1981.

[20] Kraievski NA, Smolyannikov AV, Sarkisov DS. *Pathomorphological diagnostics of human tumors. Handbook*. Moscow: Meditsina, 1993. (in Russian)

[21] Paltsev MA, Anichkov NM. *Atlas of human tumor pathology.* Moscow: Meditsina, 2005. (in Russian)

[22] Rosai J. *Rosai and Ackerman's Surgical Pathology.* Edinburgh: Mosby, 2004; pp. 515-94.

[23] Jargin SV. Pathology in the former Soviet Union: scientific misconduct and related phenomena. *Dermatol Pract Concept* 2011;1:75-81.

[24] Jargin SV. Back to Chernobyl: Some aspects of cancer diagnostics. *J Environ Stud* 2016;2(1):8.

[25] Jargin SV. Thyroid cancer after Chernobyl: obfuscated truth. *Dose Response* 2011;9(4):471-476.

[26] Chuchalin AG, Maracheva AV, Grobova OM, Cherniaev AL, Antonov NS, Kalmanova EN, Dmitrov EV, Voisin C. Lungs

exposed to nuclear catastrophe: one-year therapeutic programme in Chernobyl liquidators group. *Swiss Med Wkly* 1997;127:165-9.

[27] Degtiarova LV. A Possibility of Gastric Cancer and Malt-Lymphomas Appearance in Persons Affected because of Chernobyl Accident. *XXIII International Congress of the International Academy of Pathology and 14th World Congress of Academic and Environmental Pathology;* 15-20 October 2000; Nagoya, Japan. Pathol Int 2000; 50 Suppl. Abstract P-19-31.

[28] Derizhanova IS. The Pulmonary-Renal Syndrome among Chernobyl Nuclear Accident Liquidators. XXIII International Congress of the International Academy of Pathology and 14th World Congress of Academic and Environmental Pathology; 15-20 October 2000; Nagoya, Japan. *Pathol Int* 2000; 50 Suppl. Abstract P-19-34.

[29] Kogan EA, Cherniaev AL, Chuchalin AG, Samsonova MV, Demura SA, Sekamova SM, Zholt S, Sende B, Suanova LA, Ali-Riza AE. Morphologic and molecular-genetic characterization of lung cancer developing in people who have worked at nuclear facilities and who have lived in Russian territories polluted after the accident at the Chernobyl power plant. *Arkh Patol* 1999;61(1):22-26.

[30] Lysenko AI, Kirpatovskii ID, Pisarenko SS. Morphological changes in male sexual glands in Kaluga regions contaminated with radionuclides. *Arkh Patol* 2000;62(4):27-31.

[31] Yablokov AV, Nesterenko VB, Nesterenko AV. Chernobyl: Consequences of the catastrophe for people and the environment. *Ann N Y Acad Sci* 2009;1181.

[32] Jaworowski Z. Observations on the Chernobyl Disaster and LNT. *Dose Response* 2010;8:148-71.

[33] Iakovleva IN, Shishkov RV, Poliakov VG, Pankova PA. Clinico-morphological peculiarities of thyroid cancer among children exposed to the Chernobyl disaster radiation. *Vopr Onkol* 2008;54(3):315-20.

[34] Fridman M, Lam AK, Krasko O, Kurt Werner S, Branovan DI, et al. Morphological and clinical presentation of papillary thyroid carcinoma in children and adolescents of Belarus: the influence of

radiation exposure and the source of irradiation. *Exp Mol Pathol* 2015;98:527-31.

[35] Demidchik YE, Demidchik EP, Reiners C, Biko J, Mine M, et al. Comprehensive clinical assessment of 740 cases of surgically treated thyroid cancer in children of Belarus. *Ann Surg* 2006;243:525-32.

[36] Demidchik YE, Saenko VA, Yamashita S. Childhood thyroid cancer in Belarus, Russia, and Ukraine after Chernobyl and at present. *Arq Bras Endocrinol Metabol* 2007;51:748-62.

[37] Reiners C, Demidchik YE, Drozd VM, Biko J. Thyroid cancer in infants and adolescents after Chernobyl. *Minerva Endocrinol* 2008;33:381-95.

[38] Mamchich VI, Pogorelov AV. Surgical treatment of nodular goiter after the accident at the Chernobyl nuclear power station. *Klin Khir* 1992;(12):38-40.

[39] Demidchik IuE, Shelkovich SE. *Thyroid tumors.* Minsk: BelMAPO, 2016.

[40] Sugitani I. Management of papillary thyroid carcinoma in Japan. In: Yamashita S, Thomas G (eds) *Thyroid Cancer and Nuclear Accidents. Long-Term Aftereffects of Chernobyl and Fukushima.* London: Elsevier, 2017; pp. 185-94.

[41] La Quaglia MP, Corbally MT, Heller G, Exelby PR, Brennan MF. Recurrence and morbidity in differentiated thyroid carcinoma in children. *Surgery* 1988;104:1149-56.

[42] Danese D, Gardini A, Farsetti A, Sciacchitano S, Andreoli M, Pontecorvi A. Thyroid carcinoma in children and adolescents. *Eur J Pediatr* 1997;156:190-4.

[43] Demidchik IuE, Kontratovich VA. Repeat surgery for recurrent thyroid cancer in children. *Vopr Onkol* 2003;49(3):366-9.

[44] Arici C, Erdogan O, Altunbas H, Boz A, Melikoglu M, et al. Differentiated thyroid carcinoma in children and adolescents: clinical characteristics, treatment and outcome of 15 patients. *Horm Res* 2002;57:153-6.

[45] Giuffrida D, Scollo C, Pellegriti G, Lavenia G, Iurato MP, et al. Differentiated thyroid cancer in children and adolescents. *J Endocrinol Invest* 2002;25:18-24.

[46] Bohrer T, Pasteur I, Lyutkevych O, Fleischmann P, Tronko M. Permanent hypoparathyroidism due to thyroid cancer surgical procedures in patients exposed to radiation in the Chernobyl, Ukraine, nuclear reactor accident. *Dtsch Med Wochenschr* 2005;130:2501-6.

[47] Henry JF, Gramatica L, Denizot A, Kvachenyuk A, Puccini M, Defechereux T. Morbidity of prophylactic lymph node dissection in the central neck area in patients with papillary thyroid carcinoma. *Langenbecks Arch Surg* 1998;383(2):167-9.

[48] Contis G, Foley TP Jr. Depression, suicide ideation, and thyroid tumors among Ukrainian adolescents exposed as children to Chernobyl radiation. *J Clin Med Res* 2015;7(5):332-8.

[49] Fridman M, Savva N, Krasko O, et al. Initial presentation and late results of treatment of post-Chernobyl papillary thyroid carcinoma in children and adolescents of Belarus. *J Clin Endocrinol Metab* 2014;99(8):2932-41.

[50] Di Cristofaro J, Vasko V, Savchenko V, Cherenko S, Larin A, et al. ret/PTC1 and ret/PTC3 in thyroid tumors from Chernobyl liquidators: comparison with sporadic tumors from Ukrainian and French patients. *Endocr Relat Cancer* 2005;12:173-83.

[51] Romanenko A, Morimura K, Wei M, Zaparin W, Vozianov A, et al. DNA damage repair in bladder urothelium after the Chernobyl accident in Ukraine. *J Urol* 2002;168:973-7.

[52] Romanenko AM, Kinoshita A, Wanibuchi H, Wei M, Zaparin WK, et al. Involvement of ubiquitination and sumoylation in bladder lesions induced by persistent long-term low dose ionizing radiation in humans. *J Urol* 2006;175:739-43.

[53] Romanenko A, Kakehashi A, Morimura K, Wanibuchi H, Wei M, et al. Urinary bladder carcinogenesis induced by chronic exposure to persistent low-dose ionizing radiation after Chernobyl accident. *Carcinogenesis* 2009;30:1821-31.

[54] Romanenko A, Fukushima, S. Prediction of urinary bladder cancer induction in Ukraine after the CA. XXIII International Congress of the International Academy of Pathology and 14th World Congress of Academic and Environmental Pathology. 15-20 October 2000, Nagoya, Japan. Abstarcts. *Pathol Int* 2000;50 (Suppl):A70.

[55] Romanenko A, Morimura K, Wanibuchi H, Salim EI, Kinoshita A, et al. Increased oxidative stress with gene alteration in urinary bladder urothelium after the Chernobyl accident. Int J Cancer 2000;86:790-8.

[56] Jargin SV. Overestimation of Chernobyl consequences: biophysical aspects. *Radiat Environ Biophys 2009*;48:341-4.

[57] Romanenko A, Vozianov A, Morimura K, Fukushima S. Correspondence re: W. Paile's letter to the editor. Cancer Res., 60:1146, 2000. *Cancer Res* 2001;61:6964-5.

[58] Jargin SV. Overestimation of Chernobyl Consequences: some mechanisms. *Molodoi Uchenyi Young Sci* 2013;6:810-9.

[59] Jargin SV. Urological concern after nuclear accidents. *Urol Ann* 2018;10(3):240-2.

[60] Khmel'nitskaia NM, Orlinskaia NIu. *Complex clinico-morphological diagnostics of thyroid diseases.* St. Petersburg: Remedium Group, 2014.

[61] Jargin SV. Thyroid neoplasia after Chernobyl: a comment. *Int J Cancer* 2019;144:2897.

[62] Scott BR. It's time for a new low-dose-radiation risk assessment paradigm-one that acknowledges hormesis. Dose Response 2008;6:333-51.

[63] Jargin SV. Overestimation of Chernobyl consequences: Poorly substantiated information published. *Radiat Environ Biophys* 2010;49:743-5.

[64] Jargin SV. Unfounded statements tending to overestimate Chernobyl consequences. *J Radiol Prot* 2013;33(4):881-4.

[65] Sacks B, Meyerson G, Siegel JA. Epidemiology without biology: False paradigms, unfounded assumptions, and specious statistics in radiation science (with Commentaries by Inge Schmitz-Feuerhake and Christopher Busby and a Reply by the Authors). *Biol Theory* 2016;11:69-101.

[66] Watanabe T, Miyao M, Honda R, Yamada Y. Hiroshima survivors exposed to very low doses of A-bomb primary radiation showed a high risk for cancers. *Environ Health Prev Med* 2008;13:264-70.

Conclusion

During the 1990s, the detection of scientific misconduct seemed to be easy: plagiarism was ample (Chapters 1-5); some reports were at variance with the laws of physics [1] or principles known in medical science e.g., [2, 3]. Meanwhile, unscrupulous authors have perfected themselves in tangling and befogging their papers, making an evaluation increasingly difficult. Mutual cover-up is usual. Considering the "improvement" of fraudulent skills, scientists, editors, and authorities must jointly combat the fraudulence. Also, it is important that whistleblowers must be protected from all kinds of revenge. The response to scientific misconduct requires a national body to provide leadership and guidelines. Whistleblowers need a safe, confidential place to report scientific misconduct [4]. The quality of research and hidden conflicts of interest should be taken into account deciding which studies are to be included into reviews and meta-analyses. An international cooperation of bona fide scientists is of particular importance.

REFERENCES

[1] Jargin SV. Overestimation of Chernobyl consequences: biophysical aspects. *Radiat Environ Biophys* 2009;48(3):341-4.

[2] Jargin SV. Scientific Papers and Patents on Substances with Unproven Effects. *Recent Pat Drug Deliv Formul* 2019;13(1):37-45.

[3] Jargin SV. Scientific Papers and Patents on Substances with Unproven Effects. Part 2. *Recent Pat Drug Deliv Formul* 2019;13(3):160-73.

[4] Smith R. Research misconduct. *J R Soc Med* 2006;99(5):232-7.

About the Author

Sergei V. Jargin
Associate Professor
Peoples' Friendship University of Russia

Sergei V. Jargin graduated from the I.M. Sechenov Medical Academy in Moscow in 1983, received postgraduate training in pathology at the same institution until 1986. Thereafter, he was pathologist and lecturer at the I.M. Sechenov Medical Academy (recently renamed university). Since 1995, he has been lecturer at the Peoples' Friendship University of Russia in Moscow. His scientific interests include environmental and radiation-related pathology, renal pathology, and thyroid tumors. He is the author of more than 100 articles, books and chapters on these topics.

INDEX

A

B

C

D

E

F

G

H

I

L

M

O

P

R

S

T

U

W